Evidence-based Practice in Nursing

SAGE was founded in 1965 by Sara Miller McCune to support the dissemination of usable knowledge by publishing innovative and high-quality research and teaching content. Today, we publish over 900 journals, including those of more than 400 learned societies, more than 800 new books per year, and a growing range of library products including archives, data, case studies, reports, and video. SAGE remains majority-owned by our founder, and after Sara's lifetime will become owned by a charitable trust that secures our continued independence.

Los Angeles | London | New Delhi | Singapore | Washington DC | Melbourne

3rd Edition

Evidence-based Practice in Nursing

Peter Ellis

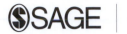

Learning Matters
An imprint of SAGE Publications Ltd
1 Oliver's Yard
55 City Road
London EC1Y 1SP

SAGE Publications Inc.
2455 Teller Road
Thousand Oaks, California 91320

SAGE Publications India Pvt Ltd
B 1/I 1 Mohan Cooperative Industrial Area
Mathura Road
New Delhi 110 044

SAGE Publications Asia-Pacific Pte Ltd
3 Church Street
#10-04 Samsung Hub
Singapore 049483

Editor: Alex Clabburn
Development editor: Richenda Milton-Daws
Production controller: Chris Marke
Project management: Swales & Willis Ltd, Exeter, Devon
Marketing manager: Tamara Navaratnam
Cover design: Wendy Scott
Typeset by: C&M Digitals (P) Ltd, Chennai, India
Printed and bound by CPI Group (UK) Ltd, Croydon, CR0 4YY

First edition published 2011
Second edition 2013
Third edition 2016

Library of Congress Control Number: 2016933145

British Library Cataloguing in Publication Data

A catalogue record for this book is available from the British Library.

ISBN 978-1-4739-1927-3
ISBN 978-1-4739-1928-0 (pbk)

At SAGE we take sustainability seriously. Most of our products are printed in the UK using FSC papers and boards. When we print overseas we ensure sustainable papers are used as measured by the PREPS grading system. We undertake an annual audit to monitor our sustainability.

Contents

Transforming Nursing Practice is a series tailor-made for pre-registration student nurses. Each book in the series is:

- ○ Affordable
- ○ Mapped to the NMC Standards and Essential Skills Clusters
- ○ Full of active learning features
- ○ Focused on applying theory to practice

Each book addresses a core topic and they have been carefully developed to be simple to use, quick to read and written in clear language.

> " An invaluable series of books that explicitly relates to the NMC standards. Each book cover a different topic that students need to explore in order to develop into a qualified nurse... I would recommend this series to all Pre-Registration nursing students whatever their field or year of study
>
> **Linda Robson**
> **Senior Lecturer, Edge Hill University**
>
> The set of books is an excellent resource for students. The series is small, easily portable and valuable. I use the whole set on a regular basis.
>
> **Fiona Davies**
> **Senior Nurse Lecturer, University of Derby**
>
> I recommend the SAGE/Learning Matters series to all my students as they are relevant and concise. Please keep up the good work.
>
> **Thomas Beary**
> **Senior Lecturer in Mental Health Nursing, University of Hertfordshire** "

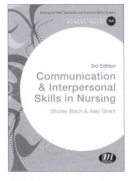

3rd Edition
Communication & Interpersonal Skills in Nursing
Shirley Bach & Alec Grant

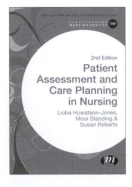

2nd Edition
Patient Assessment and Care Planning in Nursing
Lioba Howatson-Jones, Mooi Standing & Susan Roberts

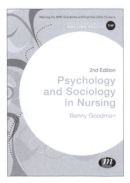

2nd Edition
Psychology and Sociology in Nursing
Benny Goodman

ABOUT THE SERIES EDITORS

Professor Shirley Bach is Head of the School of Health Sciences at the University of Brighton and responsible for the core knowledge titles. Previously she was head of post-graduate studies and has developed curriculum for undergraduate and pre-registration courses in a variety of subject domains.

Dr Mooi Standing is an Independent Academic Consultant (UK and International) and responsible for the personal and professional learning skills titles. She is an accredited NMC Quality Assurance Reviewer of educational programmes and a Professional Regulator Panellist on the NMC Practice Committee.

Sandra Walker is Senior Teaching Fellow in Mental Health at the University of Southampton and responsible for the mental health nursing titles. She is a Qualified Mental Health Nurse with a wide range of clinical experience spanning more than 20 years.

CORE KNOWLEDGE TITLES:
Becoming a Registered Nurse: Making the Transition to Practice
Communication and Interpersonal Skills in Nursing (3rd Ed)
Contexts of Contemporary Nursing (2nd Ed)
Getting into Nursing (2nd Ed)
Health Promotion and Public Health for Nursing Students (2nd Ed)
Introduction to Medicines Management in Nursing
Law and Professional Issues in Nursing (3rd Ed)
Leadership, Management and Team Working in Nursing (2nd Ed)
Learning Skills for Nursing Students
Medicines Management in Children's Nursing
Microbiology and Infection Prevention and Control for Nursing Students
Nursing and Collaborative Practice (2nd Ed)
Nursing and Mental Health Care
Nursing in Partnership with Patients and Carers
Passing Calculations Tests for Nursing Students (3rd Ed)
Palliative and End of Life Care in Nursing
Patient Assessment and Care Planning in Nursing (2nd Ed)
Patient and Carer Participation in Nursing
Patient Safety and Managing Risk in Nursing
Psychology and Sociology in Nursing (2nd Ed)
Successful Practice Learning for Nursing Students (2nd Ed)
Understanding Ethics in Nursing Practice
Using Health Policy in Nursing
What is Nursing? Exploring Theory and Practice (3rd Ed)

PERSONAL AND PROFESSIONAL LEARNING SKILLS TITLES:
Clinical Judgement and Decision Making for Nursing Students (2nd Ed)
Critical Thinking and Writing for Nursing Students (3rd Ed)
Evidence-based Practice in Nursing (3rd Ed)
Information Skills for Nursing Students
Reflective Practice in Nursing (3rd Ed)
Succeeding in Essays, Exams & OSCEs for Nursing Students
Succeeding in Literature Reviews and Research Project Plans for Nursing Students (2nd Ed)

Successful Professional Portfolios for Nursing Students (2nd Ed)
Understanding Research for Nursing Students (3rd Ed)

MENTAL HEALTH NURSING TITLES:
Assessment and Decision Making in Mental Health Nursing
Critical Thinking and Reflection for Mental Health Nursing Students
Engagement and Therapeutic Communication in Mental Health Nursing
Medicines Management in Mental Health Nursing
Mental Health Law in Nursing
Physical Healthcare and Promotion in Mental Health Nursing
Psychosocial Interventions in Mental Health Nursing

ADULT NURSING TITLES:
Acute and Critical Care in Adult Nursing (2nd Ed)
Caring for Older People in Nursing
Medicines Management in Adult Nursing
Nursing Adults with Long Term Conditions (2nd Ed)
Safeguarding Adults in Nursing Practice
Dementia Care in Nursing

You can find more information on each of these titles and our other learning resources at **www.sagepub.co.uk**. Many of these titles are also available in various e-book formats, please visit our website for more information.

Foreword

The Transforming Nursing Practice series includes several titles that focus on personal and professional learning skills needed by nurses in order to deliver safe and effective care. *Evidence-based Practice in Nursing* is a key text in this respect. The reader is encouraged to develop specific personal qualities ('dispositions of the evidence-based nurse'), including being questioning, a critical and creative thinker, reflective and reflexive, morally active, self-aware and considerate of others. The book argues that cultivating these important qualities goes hand in hand with the development and application of professional knowledge and skills in evidence-based nursing. The reader is shown how different types of evidence (research, practical knowledge/experience, health policy, patient preferences, ethical or legal issues and interprofessional feedback) can be identified, evaluated and applied to inform and enhance the quality of nursing care. The book's relevance to the practicalities of delivering high-quality, patient-centred care is highlighted in many interesting case studies. Readers' understanding of evidence-based practice in nursing is continually tested by a range of challenging learning activities. After reading this book, nursing students and others will have a good grasp of the complex nature of evidence-based practice and how they can incorporate these principles and processes to enhance the care that they give to patients.

In the third edition of this popular book the authors have incorporated changes that take account of new developments, reviewer comments and readers' feedback. It will help readers to develop current knowledge and skills in evidence-based practice and apply this to 'prioritise people – practise effectively – preserve safety – promote professionalism and trust', as required in the revised code of practise (NMC, 2015). In updating the book, the authors mirror how evidence-based practice is constantly evolving in response to new research findings, health policy and feedback from service users. This reinforces the need for lifelong learning and professional development, continually refreshing the knowledge and skills described to deliver high-quality evidence-based nursing practice.

Dr Mooi Standing
Series Editor

About the authors

Peter Ellis is the Nursing Director at Hospice in the Weald. Prior to this, Peter was a senior lecturer and programme director at Canterbury Christ Church University where he taught research and evidence-based practice, among other topics, to undergraduate and postgraduate students. Peter is also an Honorary Senior Research Fellow of Canterbury Christ Church University and has a special interest in palliative and end-of-life care.

Contributors

Dr Lioba Howatson-Jones was formerly Senior Lecturer in the School of Nursing at Canterbury Christ Church University, where she teaches pre-registration, post-registration, Master's and PhD students. Lioba's clinical nursing background is mainly in acute and radiology nursing and practice development with a particular interest in clinical supervision. Her research interests are in exploring nurses' learning and academic development.

Dr Mooi Standing is an independent nursing and educational consultant with over 40 years' experience both in the UK and internationally. In addition, she is an accredited Nursing and Midwifery Council (NMC) Quality Assurance reviewer of nursing educational programmes, and a Professional Regulator as a Panellist on the NMC Practice Committee.

Caroline Thomas is Senior Lecturer in the School of Teacher Education and Development at Canterbury Christ Church University. She is also a National Midwifery Quality Assurance Reviewer for midwifery and nursing practice.

Acknowledgements

To LHJ, thanks for the discussions which helped reform my understanding of the EBN, PE.

Introduction

One of the enduring tensions of nursing is the theory–practice gap. Some practising nurses regard this as an inevitable consequence of the move towards degree-level nursing in the UK where academics are seen as being far removed from the realities of practice while some academics regard this as being a result of practising nurses' hesitance to engage in degree-level education.

Whatever the reality of the theory–practice gap, the conscientious adoption of a coherent framework for the progression of practice through engagement with personal development and new sources of information, while maintaining a view on the realities of clinical nursing, might well help solve this dilemma.

In this book we take the view that the purpose of academic nursing is to support the enhancement of practice. To achieve this it is necessary that academic nursing takes account of the nature and realities of clinical practice. To this end we present a view of evidence-based practice that is both grounded in academic nursing (information, knowledge, evidence) and practical nursing (experience, reflection, reflexivity and patient preference). What seems clear to us in presenting this argument is that nursing is a practical undertaking and we cannot and should not engage in the creation of evidence that does not support this.

The subsequent sections will enable you to gain an overview of the messages contained within the book and how these might fit together to inform your development as an action-oriented evidence-driven nurse.

Chapter 1, Towards an inclusive model of evidence-based care: this introductory chapter sets the scene for the rest of the book and demonstrates how the various strands of evidence might be drawn together to create an inclusive picture of evidence-based nursing practice. It also examines some of the dispositions and characteristics that it might be necessary for a nurse to adopt in order to become truly evidence-based.

Chapter 2, Sources of knowledge for evidence-based care: access to information is easier now than it has ever been. The internet provides the nurse with access to sources of information that are both immediate and accessible. Newspapers, television, journals and other media carry stories about issues that affect not only health but the ways in which healthcare is delivered. The novice nurse may be tempted to use these sources of information in an unquestioning way, readily accepting what they say as being applicable to nursing practice. The more experienced nurse, or student, may feel that other sources of information are more appropriate, for instance nursing journals and professional internet-based nursing resources.

While more faith can be placed in professional sources of information, we argue in this book that there remains a need to show some caution in the sourcing and interpretation of sources of knowledge, and that even the best sources of information for practice require that the evidence-based nurse applies some criteria to judging the truth and usefulness of the information these sources contain.

Chapter 3, Critiquing research: the generic elements: any book about evidence-based practice (EBP) cannot ignore the contribution of research to the nursing evidence base. Unlike many other books about EBP, this book regards research as being of only equal importance as other sources of knowledge. Chapter 3 will explore methods for critiquing the elements of research that appear in all research papers.

Chapter 4, Critiquing research: approach-specific elements: this is a continuation of Chapter 3 and seeks to expand upon the critiquing of research that is undertaken in either the qualitative or quantitative paradigm. The appendix to this chapter, which is a critiquing framework, should be read alongside Chapters 3 and 4, as together they are intended to provide guidance of the critiquing of research for either academic purposes or to inform practice.

Chapter 5, Making sense of subjective experience: a fundamental aspect of being able to draw on many sources of information at once and to make sense of what one is hearing and seeing is having the ability to be both reflective and reflexive. Rather than explain how these strategies are practised (which is explored in the book *Reflective Practice in Nursing* in this series), Chapter 5 examines how they can contribute to our understanding of sources of evidence other than research, namely subjective knowledge.

Chapter 6, Collaborative working to achieve evidence-based care: here we explore collaborative working as a strategy for improving our evidence base for practice. The chapter explores how we as nurses can use others to develop ourselves and our understanding of care delivery. Working with others means working with different health and social care professionals (which is explored in the book *Nursing and Collaborative Practice*, also in this series) and, most importantly, patients themselves. Evidence-based practice requires nurses to be aware of, respond to and engage with the input of all individuals involved with an episode of care.

Chapter 7, Clinical decision-making in evidence-based practice: this chapter considers how the nurse might draw together various sources of evidence, reconcile the various influences on practice and apply the skills identified in earlier chapters in order to make worthwhile clinical decisions with individual patients. It challenges the reader to think about the ethical context of their decisions and how these affect individual patients, and draws together the threads of the arguments presented in the other chapters and creates a practical guide to evaluate clinical decision-making. (The issues identified in this chapter are explored in more depth in *Clinical Judgement and Decision-Making for Nursing Students*, also in this series.)

Chapter 8: Getting evidence into practice: here we explore some mechanisms by which evidence may be translated into meaningful practice. This chapter examines the social, practical and human barriers to the use of evidence in practice. It examines barriers to change and how change management strategies might be used to overcome these. It concentrates on personal and team strategies to support the adoption of evidence and what benefits might accrue from these.

NMC *Standards for Pre-registration Nursing Education* and Essential Skills Clusters

The Nursing and Midwifery Council (NMC) has standards of competence that have to be met by applicants to different parts of the nursing and midwifery register. These standards are what they deem as being necessary for the delivery of safe, effective nursing and midwifery practice.

As well as specific competencies, the NMC identifies specific skills nursing students must have at various points of their training programme. These Essential Skills Clusters (ESCs) are essential abilities that students need to attain in order to practise to their full potential.

This book includes the latest standards for 2010 onwards, taken from *Standards for Pre-registration Nursing Education* (NMC, 2010).

Learning features

Learning from reading text is not always easy. Therefore, to provide variety and to assist with the development of independent learning skills and the application of theory to practice, this book contains activities, example stories, scenarios (some with questions), case studies, concept summaries, further reading and useful websites to enable you to participate in your own learning. You will need to develop your own study skills and 'learn how to learn' to get the best from the material. The book cannot provide all the answers – but instead provides a framework for your learning.

The activities in the book will in particular help you to make sense of, and learn about, the material being presented. Some activities ask you to reflect on aspects of practice, or your experience of it, or the people or situations you encounter. *Reflection* is an essential skill in nursing, and it helps you to understand the world around you and often to identify how things might be improved. Other activities will help you develop key graduate skills such as your ability to *think critically* about a topic in order to challenge received wisdom, or your ability to *research a topic and find appropriate information and evidence*, and to be able to *make decisions* using that evidence in situations that are often difficult and time-pressured. Communication and working as part of a team are core to all nursing practice, and some activities will ask you to think about your *communication skills* to help develop these.

All the activities require you to take a break from reading the text, think through the issues presented and carry out some independent study, possibly using the internet. Where appropriate, there are sample answers presented at the end of each chapter, and these will help you to understand more fully your own reflections and independent study. You will gain most from the activities if you try to complete them yourself before reading the suggested answers. Remember, academic study will always require independent work; attending lectures will never be enough to be successful on your programme, and these activities will help to deepen your knowledge and understanding of the issues under scrutiny and give you practice at working on your own.

You might want to think about completing these activities as part of your personal development plan (PDP) or portfolio. After completing the activity write it up in your PDP or portfolio in a section devoted to that particular skill, then look back over time to see how far you have developed. You can also do more of the activities for a key skill that you have identified a weakness in, which will help build your skill and confidence in this area.

There is a glossary of terms at the end of the book that provides an interpretation of some of the terminology in the context of the subject of the book. Glossary terms are in bold in the first instance that they appear.

All chapters have further reading and useful websites listed at the end, with notes to show you why we think they will be helpful to you. The websites will also help you to remain up to date with developments in this aspect of practice as awareness of key issues grows and policies develop.

We hope that you find this book helpful in developing your professional practice and that it challenges you to ensure you provide care and support that reduces the risk of vulnerability and promotes dignity, respect and a positive quality of life.

Chapter 1
Towards an inclusive model of evidence-based care

Peter Ellis

NMC Standards for Pre-registration Nursing Education

This chapter will address the following competencies:

Domain 3: Nursing practice and decision-making

1. All nurses must use up-to-date knowledge and evidence to assess, plan, deliver and evaluate care, communicate findings, influence change and promote health and best practice. They must make person-centred, evidence-based judgements and decisions, in partnership with others involved in the care process, to ensure high-quality care. They must be able to recognise when the complexity of clinical decisions requires specialist knowledge and expertise, and consult or refer accordingly.

5. All nurses must understand public health principles, priorities and practice in order to recognise and respond to the major causes and social determinants of health, illness and health inequalities. They must use a range of information and data to assess the needs of people, groups, communities and populations, and work to improve health, well-being and experiences of healthcare; secure equal access to health screening, health promotion and healthcare; and promote social inclusion.

NMC Essential Skills Clusters

This chapter will address the following ESCs:

Cluster: Care, compassion and communication

1. As partners in the care process, people can trust a newly registered graduate nurse to provide collaborative care based on the highest standards, knowledge and competence.

2. People can trust the newly registered graduate nurse to engage in person centred care empowering people to make choices about how their needs are met when they are unable to meet them for themselves.

8. People can trust the newly registered graduate nurse to gain their consent based on sound understanding and informed choice prior to any intervention and that their rights in decision-making and consent will be respected and upheld.

continued …

Cluster: Organisational aspects of care

12. People can trust the newly registered graduate nurse to respond to their feedback and a wide range of other sources to learn, develop and improve services.

Chapter aims

After reading this chapter, you will be able to:

- understand that evidence for practice comes in many forms;
- identify key components of the evidence base for practice;
- understand why evidence for practice is important;
- begin to create a coherent picture of what critical practice actually means.

Introduction

Nurses work in ever-changing environments of care. Changes in governmental and local policy, improvements in technology and pharmaceuticals, the changing demography of the world and developments in society all impact on the ways in which we deliver care to patients. Not only do we face the challenge of a constantly changing and evolving workplace, but as a student nurse you have to try to make sense of what you learn in the classroom and how this relates to the realities of what you experience in the workplace. As a staff nurse the pressures increase somewhat as you continue to work in an ever-changing environment, one that requires you to evolve and develop with it in order to deliver high-quality care, for which you are now professionally accountable.

All of the pressures of care delivery can lead to an overwhelming feeling of helplessness. Perhaps you feel that you might not know all you think you should know before you go on to the wards, or that what you have learnt might well be out of date soon. Being prepared for life as a nurse requires you to embrace the many opportunities for lifelong learning so you can develop skills in identifying and evaluating information (evidence) that will stand you in good stead through-out your nursing career.

This chapter seeks to set the scene for the rest of the book in describing an attitude and approach to learning and development that will help support you, as a student or trained nurse, in making sense of where you work and what you do in practice. It is the aim of this chapter to stimulate you to think about how and why you practise in the way you do and how you can make sense of the various influences on your practice.

This approach might seem at odds with an evidence-based practice approach to care; after all, isn't evidence all about being able to access, critique and apply research to practice? Of course to some extent this is right, but in this book we take the view that research is not the only source of knowledge for practice – nor should it be.

We argue that, in order to truly act in an evidential way in practice, the nurse needs to knit together many sources of evidence. The position we take is that sources of knowledge may stand alone as evidence, or may serve to validate or refute other sources of evidence. For example, a randomised controlled trial may demonstrate the worth of a 'keep fit' intervention for weight loss, and this evidence may be validated by a qualitative enquiry that shows that the people involved enjoy the keep fit and want to do it. Conversely, they may not enjoy the process and therefore the intervention will ultimately fail.

In this book we demonstrate that all the different sources of information and influences on the way in which nursing is practised are potentially of equal importance at one time or another. We further show that to nurse effectively in the twenty-first century, and beyond, requires you to be able to identify and use all forms of information in order to turn them into evidence that will be used to inform practice.

In order to achieve this, this chapter explores some of the influences that have shaped nursing practice. It describes and explores the rise of evidence-based practice and develops a big-picture view of how you can prepare yourself for the challenges of modern practice. Rising to this challenge requires you to adopt a constantly questioning approach to your practice that is both beneficial to your learning and working life, and, ultimately and importantly, to your patients – that is to be a truly evidential practitioner you need to adopt a questioning and reflective attitude to your work.

Activity 1.1   *Reflection*

Try to remember what made you want to study to become a nurse in the first place. Stop and think about what you thought would inform and guide what you would do in your everyday practice as a nurse before you became a nursing student. Talk to others on your programme about what they felt or thought about this.

As this activity is based on your own observation, there is no outline answer at the end of the chapter.

The likely feeling you will have about Activity 1.1 is that your practice would be guided by the people who teach you and those who work with you in practice. Of course, this is widely the case, but there are a few issues with the apprenticeship model of nurse education in that it can propagate outdated or even poor practice. Sometimes teachers and mentors do not know the answers to questions, and even if they do, learning to be dependent on others for information and understanding is not the best way to prepare for life as a nurse who is autonomous and evidence-based. So clearly developing a sense of the need for evidence to guide your own practice and the ability to identify and apply it early on in your career is no bad thing.

Why evidence-based nursing is important

There is a culture of increasing scrutiny of the work of health and social care professionals which has come about, at least in part, in response to various scandals (see the case studies in the box below). Such public scandals have contributed to a climate of care in which nurses are increasingly required to be able to justify the decisions they make with and for patients. No longer is it good enough for nurses to claim they know what is best for their patients just because they are nurses. The rise in patient power and the governmental agenda of service user consultation and involvement (Department of Health (DH), 1989, 1991, 2001, 2012a; National Institute for Health and Care Excellence (NICE), 2011, 2012) have created a climate of care in which nurses have to be able to justify not only what they do but also how and why they are doing it.

Case study: Some of the scandals that have affected healthcare in the UK

On 25 February 2000, Victoria Climbié died after years of neglect and abuse from her aunt and aunt's boyfriend. In his report of the inquiry into the death of Victoria, Lord Laming states: I found it hard to understand why established good medical practice, that would have undoubtedly helped clarify the complexities in Victoria's case, was not followed.

*In January 2001 the Redfern report criticised the actions of a pathologist at the children's hospital, Alder Hey, for removing and retaining human organs and tissue samples without consent. The public outcry that followed led the UK government to publish new guidelines outlining the law on the handling of human body parts (****www.rlcinquiry.org.uk****).*

On 15 April 2009 Margaret Haywood was struck off the Nursing and Midwifery Council's register for secretly filming the alleged neglect of elderly patients at the Royal Sussex Hospital. The public response to the programme had been one of outrage.

In 2013 the Francis report into the failings at Mid Staffordshire NHS Foundation Trust made some important observations about the failure of care within the Trust:

The negative aspects of culture in the system were identified as including:

- a lack of openness to criticism;
- a lack of consideration for patients;
- defensiveness;
- looking inwards not outwards;
- secrecy;
- misplaced assumptions about the judgements and actions of others;
- an acceptance of poor standards;
- a failure to put the patient first in everything that is done.

This report became one of the key drivers for change in care provision in the UK.

There is no doubting that nursing takes place very much in the public eye, and when nurses and other health and social care professionals make mistakes, they come in for severe criticism. There is also without a doubt a feeling in society at large that all care professionals should know what they are doing, why they are doing it and do it well.

Such expectations are daunting but very understandable, and most nurses aspire to live up to these very reasonable expectations. Clearly, knowledge of what evidence-based practice is will not be sufficient for you to meet these expectations; however, knowledge of how you might go about identifying evidence to inform practice and how you might subsequently assimilate this evidence into your practice will be. In short, evidence-based nursing practice is not a purely academic exercise; it is a means of knitting together knowledge from a number of different sources in a way that has the potential to impact positively on what we do as nurses: care.

Activity 1.2 — *Reflection*

Think about a time that you, or a family member, were a patient. How well do you feel you were kept informed about the care you received and why it was being delivered in the way it was? Ask a more experienced colleague what it was like to be a nurse in the past and how the evidence-based care agenda has changed the way in which care is delivered. Do they think it is a good thing or a bad thing? Why?

An outline of what you might find is given at the end of the chapter.

Knowing what you are doing and why informs part of an important element of modern nursing and healthcare practice called **clinical governance**. Clinical governance is a system whereby what nurses, and other care professionals, do in practice is subjected to scrutiny to ensure it is worthwhile and money is being spent wisely. NICE and National Service Frameworks (NSFs) create guidelines and policies about how National Health Service (NHS) money is used. They use evidence from many sources to inform the policies they produce, and these are widely regarded as guides to good practice.

Activity 1.3 — *Evidence-based practice and research*

Have a look at some NICE guidelines on a subject you know something about. Pay particular attention to what evidence informed the decision-making and who was involved in drawing up the guidance. Consider how you might gather the information you might need to answer the same question and whether you consider the approach taken by NICE to be comprehensive and reasonable.

The website address for NICE is given at the end of the chapter in the Useful websites section.

As this activity is based on your own observation, there is no outline answer at the end of the chapter.

Not only is the requirement to evidence what we do as nurses a result of political and social pressure, but there are good moral reasons as to why nurses need to show that what they are doing is in the best interests of their patients. Accountability is a central tenet of the Nursing and Midwifery Council's Code (2015), which states that nurses must:

> *Always practise in line with the best available evidence … To achieve this, you must:*

> **6.1** *make sure that any information or advice given is evidence-based, including information relating to using any healthcare products or services, and*

> **6.2** *maintain the knowledge and skills you need for safe and effective practice.*

Beauchamp and Childress (2013) argue that ethical practice in healthcare requires that the providers of care, including nurses and student nurses, are mindful of what they term the four principles of healthcare ethics. These are:

- beneficence (doing good);
- non-maleficence (avoiding unnecessary harm);
- autonomy (respecting freedom of action);
- justice (fairness).

There are, of course, a number of other ethical approaches that might inform how we act as nurses, but the message from Beauchamp and Childress has clear connections as to why evidence is important in nursing.

The other school of ethical thought that might inform practice is that of consequentialism (doing things that have the best outcomes); the nurse might select a course of action with his or her patient that is perceived to have the highest probability of achieving the desired outcome of care.

In the UK, we are used to the idea that healthcare is provided 'free at the point of use'; indeed, this is one of the founding principles of the National Health Service, and one of the things that makes it such a special institution in which people hold great pride. However, 'free at the point of use' is not the same as 'free'. The money that funds the activity of the NHS comes directly out of the public purse; it is money that is raised through taxation and national insurance contributions and, as such, it is money that needs to be spent wisely. There are many pressures on how NHS money is used, and to spend money on futile practices means that there is less money available elsewhere in the system for other things. The use of evidence in practice is therefore essential in order to help make the money available go as far as it can reasonably be expected to. The idea of getting good value for money links strongly to the concepts of ethics and governance discussed above.

Some of the reasons why adopting an evidential approach to nursing is important are:

- accountability to our professional body;
- it improves the likelihood of good quality outcomes of care;
- professionalism of nursing;

- governance;
- it shows good use of resources;
- moral and ethical imperatives;
- to improve clients' lives;
- it helps us plan effective interventions.

Recent developments in nursing and in healthcare in general – for example, the increase in advanced nurse practitioner and nurse consultant roles as well as the move from hospital to community-based care – have had a dramatic impact on the ways in which nurses practise. The need for an increase in autonomous working while supporting and developing interprofessional and patient-centred approaches to care means that the nurse is required *to always practise in line with the best available evidence* (NMC, 2015). Such decision-making requires nurses to be familiar with the most current evidence and how this applies to the situations that arise in their practice.

Traditionally, nursing practice was built on an apprenticeship model whereby students learnt to nurse in a manner that reflected what was deemed to represent good nursing by the ward sister and the staff nurses on duty. As such, the way in which nursing care was delivered was based on historical ways of working that had been passed down between generations of nurses with little change and little in the way of questioning. Such practices can become ritualised and are practised because 'that is what we have always done'. Not all nursing traditions are bad or detrimental; for example, the regular changing of linen and bedding – at one time more a matter of pleasing matron than anything else – is now known to play a role in infection control. However, some traditions are at odds with the notions of evidence-based practice that are presented in this book primarily because they are undertaken in an unquestioning and unthinking way.

In this section we have identified that there are a number of reasons why evidence-based practice for nursing is essential. We have seen that adopting evidence-informed ways of working is not an optional extra that nurses can ignore if they are too busy. Key among the reasons for adopting a questioning and evidence-based approach to care provision are the ethical arguments about doing good and avoiding harm, the wise use of resources and the development of nursing as a more autonomous profession. In the next section we will examine what evidence-based practice might actually mean.

Definitions of evidence-based practice

There has been – and there remains – some debate about what evidence-based practice actually means. There are many definitions of evidence-based practice, research-informed practice, evidence-based medicine, evidence-based healthcare and evidence-based nursing in the literature. Before we go on to define what we mean by evidence-based practice in this book, and before we explore the concepts that might inform such practice for nursing, it is worth exploring some of these definitions in an attempt to get a feel for what EBP might actually be.

The number and diversity of the definitions demonstrate that there is little agreement between professionals within healthcare as to what exactly evidence-based care means. This can be a source of confusion for the student nurse, who should take time to reflect upon what they thought nursing practice was based on before they started nursing, once they started nursing and again as they become more familiar with nursing practice.

Polit and Beck (2008, p3) define evidence-based practice as:

> *the use of best clinical evidence in making patient care decisions … such evidence typically comes from research conducted by nurses and other health care professionals.*

This definition places research squarely at the centre of **clinical decision-making** and recognises that such research may come from sources other than just the nursing profession.

Perhaps the most widely quoted definition comes from Sackett et al. (1996, p71), who defined evidence-based medicine as:

> *the conscientious, explicit and judicious use of current best evidence in making decisions about the care of the individual patient. It means integrating individual clinical expertise with the best available external clinical evidence from systematic research.*

This definition identifies a number of important markers of evidence-based practice.

- It is conscientious – it is a purposeful activity one chooses to engage in.
- It is explicit – it is applied in such a way that it can be shown to have been used.
- It is judicious – thought has been given to how it applies to the job in hand.
- It is about the care of the individual patient – the evidence fits the situation one is dealing with.
- It is a mix of individual expertise with knowledge that has been gathered from good quality research.

What Sackett et al. are saying is that one answer will not fit all clinical scenarios and that it is the role of the doctor, in this case, to identify the research that best fits the clinical situation that is in front of them. McKibbon (1998, p399) provides a more far-reaching and inclusive definition.

> *Evidence-based practice (EBP) is an approach to health care wherein health professionals use the best evidence possible, i.e. the most appropriate information available, to make clinical decisions for individual patients. EBP values, enhances and builds on clinical expertise, knowledge of disease mechanisms, and pathophysiology. It involves complex and conscientious decision-making based not only on the available evidence but also on patient characteristics, situations, and preferences. It recognizes that health care is individualized and ever changing and involves uncertainties and probabilities. Ultimately EBP is the formalization of the care process that the best clinicians have practised for generations.*

This explanation of EBP goes beyond the other two definitions in recognising the importance of the patient in making decisions ('preferences') about their own care and, as such, perhaps better reflects modern nursing practice incorporating person-centred care.

If we are to move the concept of EBP in nursing forward, it is perhaps best to attach it to well-established, patient-focused strategies with which nurses are all familiar. The nursing process of assessing, planning, implementing and evaluating care can be seen to be similar to the stages of implementing EBP that Moule (2015) suggests.

1. Identify a problem from practice and turn it into a specific question.

2. Find the best available evidence that relates to the question, usually by systematically searching the literature.

3. Appraise the evidence.

4. Identify the best evidence alongside the patient's needs and preferences.

5. Evaluate the effect of applying the evidence.

Stage 1 reflects the assessment process in nursing during which the problem to be addressed is identified and framed. Stages 2, 3 and 4 involve a conscientious and explicit planning phase during which the evidence that will underpin the plan is identified and assessed, and the patient's circumstances and preferences are accounted for. This is followed by the implementation of the plan, and the evaluation of the effectiveness of what has been done in the final stage of the nursing process and stage 5 of Moule's (2015) framework.

What is apparent from all these definitions and the application of the nursing process is that EBP is a framework for action and not academic debate and, as such, it places EBP squarely at the heart of nursing practice.

Activity 1.4   *Reflection*

Which definition of EBP do you best identify with? What is it about the definition which captures your attention and makes you think this is the right definition? Using the information presented in this section and your own experience to date, write your own definition of evidence-based practice.

As this activity is based on your own observations, there is no outline answer at the end of the chapter.

The approach to the use of EBP is mirrored in the widely cited Critical Appraisal Skills Programme (CASP; see Useful websites). CASP asks two important and related questions: how do I know a piece of research has been undertaken properly and that its findings are reliable, and when different research points to different answers how do I know which to believe? The CASP initiative is designed to help care professionals get evidence into practice in three key stages:

1. find the evidence;
2. appraise the evidence;
3. act on the evidence.

This approach mirrors the approach of this book: Chapter 2 tells us how to find evidence from good sources; Chapters 3 and 4 give examples of how to critique research and Chapters 7 and 8 demonstrate how to put evidence into practice. Find, appraise and act is a good mantra for evidence-based nursing practice. Of course, as with the nursing process, the final stage of the implantation of a plan is to evaluate effectiveness – this is where reflection becomes important for the second time on the EBP cycle (see Chapter 5).

Hierarchies of evidence

This consideration of what evidence-based nursing practice is leads to an important question: if we are to evaluate the research evidence, how do we know which form of research evidence is best and consequently what we should do in practice?

Answering the question 'Which form of research evidence is best?' requires us to do two things. First, we need to understand which forms of evidence are regarded as the strongest. Second, we need to be able to evaluate individual pieces of research, identifying their strengths and weaknesses, and thereby coming to some conclusion about how good the individual piece of research is. Information on how to address this second step will be covered in more detail in Chapters 3 and 4. Here we will turn our attention to the first step.

As with the definitions of EBP, there is little agreement between different professions and individual practitioners as to what constitutes good evidence. This may be surprising to the novice nurse who assumes that everyone knows what they are doing and why they are doing it. In order to understand why there are differences in opinion it is worth remembering that there are many different types of question that arise in nursing practice, and that these relate not only to the provision of specific care but also to how the care is experienced and the relationships between individuals giving and receiving care (see Chapters 3 and 4 for the types of research that are used to answer specific questions from practice). For now we should consider what is termed the hierarchy of evidence, more often presented as the hierarchy of research evidence.

Hierarchies of evidence give the practitioner and researcher alike some insight into the perceived worth of individual approaches to research. The classic hierarchy of research evidence is given in Table 1.1. It takes account only of **quantitative research** methods and does not allow for **qualitative research** methods or clinical experience or opinion.

Polit and Beck (2008, p ii) present a perhaps more useful hierarchy of evidence. This gives some weighting to evidence that takes account of qualitative research as a source of evidence as well as valuing experience and practice expertise, and other evidence that is not research based (see Table 1.2). This hierarchy is more in line with the concept of evidence that is presented in this book.

	Level	Description
Table 1.1: Example of a classic hierarchy of research evidence		
Strongest	1	Meta analyses and systematic reviews – reviews of multiple research reports and the statistics within them.
	2	Randomised controlled trials with definitive results – clinical trials that involve a new intervention that is assessed against another established intervention or no intervention at all and that show a definite result.
	3	Randomised controlled trials with non-definitive results – clinical trials which involve a new intervention which is assessed against another established intervention or no intervention at all which show a probable result.
	4	Prospective cohort studies/outcomes studies – long-term follow-up studies of large groups of people usually in their natural setting.
	5	Case-control studies – backward-looking studies that demonstrate associations between causes of disease and diseases or other causes and effects.
	6	Cross-sectional studies – studies undertaken in one period in time that measure potential cause and effect simultaneously.
Weakest	7	Case reports – clinical reports of individual episodes of care.

Based on the work of Petticrew and Roberts (2003).

Activity 1.5   *Critical thinking*

The NMC's generic standard for competence for nursing practice and decision-making states that: *All practice should be informed by the best available evidence and comply with local and national guidelines* (NMC, 2010, p17). Do you think that either of the hierarchies of evidence presented above enables you to do this?

There are some possible answers and thoughts at the end of the chapter.

Hierarchies of evidence give the busy nurse some idea as to the level of trust they should place in an individual research methodology or review paper. What hierarchies don't do is answer

	Level	Description
Table 1.2: Polit and Beck's hierarchy of research evidence		
Strongest	1	(a) Systematic review of randomised controlled trials (RCTs); (b) systematic review of non-randomised trials – reviews of clinical experiments that are undertaken using: (i) comparable groups; or (ii) non-comparable groups.
	2	(a) Single RCT; (b) single non-randomised trial – (i) one experimental clinical study; (ii) one non-experimental clinical study.
	3	Systematic review of correlational/observational studies – reviews of studies that examine associations between causes and effects.
	4	Single correlational/observational study – one study that examines associations between causes and effects.
	5	Systematic review of descriptive/qualitative/physiologic studies – reviews of studies that only describe an event or experience or that measure individual biological variables.
	6	Single descriptive/qualitative/physiologic study – studies that only describe an event or experience or that measure individual biological variables.
Weakest	7	Opinions of authorities/expert committees – collections of the understanding and interpretations of people who are experienced in a given area.

Based on the work of Polit and Beck (2008).

questions about the quality of an individual piece of research (see Chapters 3 and 4) nor do they give any indication as to how to deal with an individual patient or clinical question. This is because not all research undertaken using strong research methodologies is itself good quality and because we cannot assume the findings of a piece of research will apply to all patients who are broadly similar to those involved in the research.

In Chapter 2 issues of the identification of sources of research evidence are addressed in some detail. It is perhaps sufficient at this stage to have made the point that not all evidence is regarded as equal and that we should be aware that value judgements need to be made when thinking about the types of research evidence we choose to inform our nursing practice. We should also remember that not all evidence for nursing practice is gained from research, and that there are elements of experience and reflection that also need to be accounted for, as we shall see in Chapter 5. We must also be aware that nursing is a person-centred activity and as such the application of evidence must take into account issues of policy, resources, expertise and the individual patient's situation and personal preferences.

On reviewing the hierarchies of evidence you may have noticed that **systematic reviews** appear as the top layer in both examples. Systematic reviews (together with **meta-analyses**) use the data from multiple studies to gain a bigger, and more robust, understanding of a clinical issue. Think of systematic reviews as a means of gathering all the outcomes of similar studies examining similar issues and merging them all together so that the weaknesses associated with any single study become diluted and the shared strengths of the various studies combine to allow a clear answer to a clinical question to emerge. Systematic reviews include and exclude studies according to very rigid and objective criteria; they assess the quality of the evidence before it is included and provide robust reasons for what they are doing. In this sense systematic reviews are exactly as described: they are systematic in the application of inclusion and exclusion criteria and in applying criteria to the quality reviewing of existing studies.

We do not explain how to undertake or critique a systematic review in this book, but some useful sources of further information are to be found at the end of the chapter. Perhaps the most famous source for systematic clinical reviews is the Cochrane database, which contains in excess of 5000 reviews of clinical evidence. Systematic reviews should not be confused with simple reviews, as in many review articles. Plain reviews do not necessarily apply any criteria to the search for, nor appraisal of, the literature they include and, in this sense, cannot therefore be said to be *systematic*.

While systematic reviews might sit at the top of the hierarchies of evidence, they do take account of individual circumstances and preferences and so, alongside all of the influences on evidence-based nursing practice, they are a necessary, but not sufficient, individual influence for practice decisions. In the next section of this chapter, we will consider how the various strands of influence might come together in a meaningful way in order to advance nursing practice.

Advancing the meaning of evidence

Typically, the greatest impacts on individual nursing practice are the clinical lessons learnt as students, and indeed, once qualified, the lessons learnt from our nursing and other professional peers. Prior to the explosion of evidence-based practice, the ward sister and the matron dictated the ways in which the nurses worked in their departments and on their wards. This 'sister knows best' working ethos still has a pervasive impact on contemporary nursing practice.

What you learn in the classroom, away from practice, often seems remote and unrelated to the realities of high turn-over, stressful nursing practice (Pijl-Zieber et al., 2015). Sometimes lessons learnt appear to be right in the classroom, but lose their appeal in the cold light of the practice environment. At other times it is easier to choose not to discuss or implement such lessons in order to avoid 'rocking the boat' or appearing to be a troublemaker – you might think it is perhaps best to wait until you are in charge to implement what you know to be right. The conflict between what we 'know' and what we do is a source of anxiety for many nurses and student nurses.

In part, this book lays down a challenge to all nurses, including students, to think about the ethics of what they do and how they do it. It challenges us not only to know what is right but also to practise in a way that is justifiable.

Clearly, this is a hard thing to ask of any nurse, let alone a student nurse. The question remains, however: if you would want to know the rationale for what someone is doing to you, why would you not provide a rationale for the care that you are providing to someone else? Elsewhere in this series (Ellis, 2014) we make the argument that ethics is everyone's business and that nurses should take responsibility for the choices and the actions they undertake.

This chapter has so far established that EBP is not an exclusively research-driven ideal but more a way of working and questioning (what we refer to as 'attitude and approach to learning and development' earlier in this chapter), and drawing on sources of knowledge to continuously evolve practice. We have demonstrated that EBP is important for a number of very good reasons and we have come to some conclusions about what EBP is.

It is important at this point to say that there are a number of skills you can learn and attitudes you can adopt in order to develop EBP in your own practice. Unlike most books on evidence-based practice, this book seeks to explore and develop the skills that you need to continue to develop as a nurse who practises in an evidence-driven, patient-focused manner. In order to develop these skills you need to recognise the influences on your thinking and learning, and hence on the way in which you practise. Common influences on how you practise include: what you have been taught in your training; research you have read; experiences you have had; experience of others that you have listened to (including those of patients, nurses and other professionals); local and national policies; pressure from managers; and ethical considerations and social norms.

With all of these influences on your practice it is necessary that you learn to treat each situation as a learning experience; that is, that you are willing to learn from and apply learning to each new situation you encounter. This learning is not just about believing what you are told or what you read; it is about being critical about what you learn and experience, appraising it, considering its usefulness and seeing how it marries up with what you already know (or think you know).

One famous nursing theorist, Carper (1978), identified four ways of 'knowing' in nursing. She labelled these empirical, aesthetic, ethical and personal knowledge (an explanation of each of

Table 1.3: Carper's ways of 'knowing' in nursing practice	
Way of knowing	**Meaning**
Empirical knowledge	Knowledge found in textbooks or journal papers that is derived from research and that is provable.
Aesthetic knowledge	Subjective and unique knowledge that requires interpretation, creativity, empathy, understanding and valuing. It is knowledge that feels and looks right.
Ethical knowledge	Knowledge based on systems of belief and moral codes of conduct.
Personal knowledge	Knowledge that arises out of experience as sympathy, empathy and understanding.
Based on the work of Carper (1978).	

these is given in Table 1.3). Taken together, Carper suggests that these sources of knowledge give us the 'evidence' on which to base nursing practice.

We have established that there are a number of important influences on the way in which nursing is practised and that there are a range of forms of knowledge that might be used to inform nursing practice. What is needed now is a scheme by which we can draw all these elements together and make sense of not only sources of evidence but also influences on nursing practice.

Developing as an evidence-based nurse

Brechin (2000, p25) presents three pillars for what she calls 'critical practice'; these are presented in Table 1.4. These pillars are tools the nurse can employ to develop an inclusive model of practice, one that recognises the need to want to do what is best for the patient while acting in a manner that respects and includes all the individuals involved, especially the patient; as the Code puts it to *recognise and respect the contribution that people can make to their own health and well-being* (NMC, 2015). These pillars, or ways of working, require that even as the nurse becomes more practised and knowledgeable in what they do, they take on board and adapt this knowledge in the light of new information, evidence and individual circumstances.

Brechin's pillars tell us something about the sort of person that is needed and the attitude to care that is required of the evidence-based nurse. They support the notions that were advanced earlier in the chapter – that becoming an evidence-based nurse is about making a positive difference and that this difference has to be made in conjunction with our patients and other staff.

Table 1.4: Brechin's pillars of critical practice

Pillar	What this might mean	Example
Forging relationships	Working with others.	Being open and honest in communication.
Seeking to empower others	Giving back control.	Seeking to support patient choices.
Making a difference	Improving something.	Playing a part in helping someone recover from illness.

Based on the work of Brechin (2000).

Barnett (2000) claims that professional life now requires more than the handling of mere complexity (i.e. managing overwhelming data and theories). It is also about handling multiple frames of reference – a condition he calls supercomplexity. Supercomplexity might arise in nursing practice when the nurse is required to pay attention not only to the realities of a patient's condition and its treatment (Carper's empirical knowledge) but also to the patient's circumstances and wishes (aesthetic knowledge), the policies and practices of the hospital, their own values and moral codes (ethical knowledge) and their own previous experiences of delivering care to someone in a similar position or with the same disease (personal knowledge).

Barnett (2000) asserts that the main teaching task of a higher education institute should not just be to transmit knowledge but should be to develop in students the attributes appropriate to conditions of supercomplexity. It is the intention of this book to signpost and start to explore some of these attributes and present you, the reader, with options for self-development that will enable you to embrace a life of learning, development and evidenced care giving.

In order to achieve this state whereby one is able to function within supercomplex systems, Barnett claims that you must embrace three dimensions of being: knowledge, self-identity and action. These three elements of making sense of a complex workplace reflect quite well the central arguments of this book and this chapter – that evidence-based practice is about:

- knowledge (perhaps research based);
- working with others (especially patients); and
- the delivery of care (that is, EBP is about action and not just words).

A model of evidence-based nursing

The model of evidence-based nursing on which this book is based is one of informed nursing action delivered with an understanding and appreciation of the complexity not only of the information associated with the medical management of a patient but also of the complex nature of human interaction, beliefs and ethics. Figure 1.1 presents some of the influences on the nurse practising in an evidence-based manner. It shows some of the attributes and skills that need to be developed in order to become an evidence-based nurse and illustrates that all action has to take account of ethical and moral practice.

The rest of the book is given over to examining and explaining these various skills, sources and knowledge. Taken together, they form one proposal for how you might develop to become, and continue to be, an evidence-based nurse.

Activity 1.6   *Critical thinking*

Adopting the questioning approach to practice (see Figure 1.1), which embraces and juggles many seemingly competing sources of knowledge, while adopting some positive personal attributes or dispositions (characteristics) advocated in Figure 1.1, is seemingly a hard task. There appear to be a large number of things that the nurse needs to do in order to engage with this model. This is certainly true.

Now reflect on your own personal and professional behaviours and orientations to nursing practice. For example, why did you become a nurse and what was it that you thought you

---

continued ...

might achieve by taking on this role? Which of the attributes do you already possess? Which of these attributes would you like to develop? Can you see any connections between the dispositions? Are there some that you think complement each other?

An outline of what you might find is given at the end of the chapter.

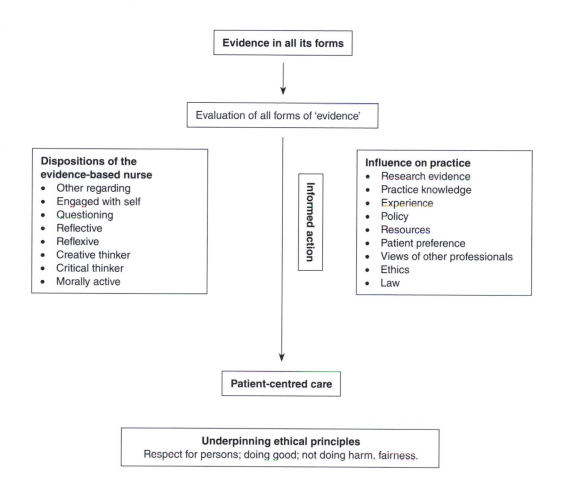

Figure 1.1: The influences on and dispositions of an evidence-based nurse

You may have formed the impression during your training or time on the wards that evidence-based practice was really only a term that academics used to disguise modules about research. The main message of the book is that evidence-based practice is about using various forms of information – not just research – to guide and develop practice.

continued ...

In this chapter we have seen that identifying and adopting evidence for practice is a multi-stage process that requires discovering sources of potential knowledge and then asking questions about the quality of the information found.

We have identified and demonstrated that EBP is about practice and not just words. It is about what we do and how we can know that what we are doing in clinical practice is the right thing to do. We have seen that evidence takes many forms and that there are a number of skills and attitudes to learning that need to be adopted by the nurse in order to support the creation and adoption of evidence-based practice.

This chapter has established that nurses need to identify high-quality sources of knowledge for practice and that they need to take account of the quality of the information that these sources present. It has shown that to be a successful evidence-based nurse, one has to engage in lifelong learning and adopt a questioning approach to one's practice. This chapter has discussed the need to involve the patient and other professionals in decision-making about the patient's care and the fact that research evidence alone does not always provide sufficient grounds on which to base clinical decision-making and action.

Activities: Brief outline answers

Activity 1.2: Reflection (page 9)

There is a clear link between our ability as nurses to explain to our patients what we are doing and our ability to explain why. All too often nurses are involved in care but do not understand the rationale behind what they are doing. This will mean that the information passed to patients (in which I include myself and family members) is about what is going to happen and not why or how this will help. Over the last 20 or 30 years there has been a growing acceptance among nurses that this is no longer an acceptable way to practise and that as nurses we need to be able to justify what we do in practice to – and, indeed, with – our patients and clients.

Activity 1.5: Critical thinking (page 15)

The hierarchies of evidence allow us to make judgements about the likely usefulness of competing forms of evidence in our planning and delivery of care. They suggest quite strongly that some forms of evidence are better than others at informing what we might do and how we do it. Clearly, as with all elements of evidence-based practice, the findings of research need to be interpreted alongside the patient's situation, the skills and resources available, and the patient's preference. We also need to remain cognisant of the fact that even high-quality research methodologies can be poorly applied and therefore individual studies may not be as useful as they might otherwise be.

Activity 1.6: Critical thinking (page 20)

What appears clear from the dispositions of the evidence-based nurse is that there are a number of important links between some attributes, such as: 'other regarding' and 'morally active'; 'questioning' and 'critical thinker'; and 'engaged with self' and 'reflective'. The development of a more structured approach to questioning, as derived from critical thinking, will also feed into the individual nurse becoming more questioning in general; while adopting a more other focused way of thinking will certainly add something to the nurse's ability to think morally and ethically.

It is probably true that you entered nursing to make a difference to the lives of patients and that you are reading this book because you think it might enhance your ability to do so. This demonstrates that you may already have attributes that include being 'other regarding', questioning and reflective. Learning to see how all of these dispositions come together to create and enhance evidence-based practice is therefore only a matter of consciously engaging with the process of consolidating, developing and exploring the links between attributes that you already have while being open to cultivating new attributes to complement them.

Further reading

Aveyard, H (2010) *Doing a literature review in health and social care: a practical guide* (2nd edn). Maidenhead: Open University Press.

A clear introductory guide to literature reviewing.

Fink, A (2010) *Conducting research literature reviews: from the internet to paper* (3rd edn.) London: Sage.

A more advanced book about literature reviews.

Gerrish, K and Lathlean, J (2015) *The research process in nursing* (7th edn). Oxford: Wiley-Blackwell.

Especially Chapter 38. This chapter examines what evidence-based practice might look like.

Gomm, R and Davies, C (eds) (2000) *Using evidence in health and social care.* London: Sage.

Especially Chapters 1 and 7. These chapters examine the different ways in which we can know things and how we can get evidence into practice.

Moule, P (2015) *Making sense of research in nursing, health and social care* (5th edn). London: Sage.

Especially Chapters 1 and 2. These chapters explore the role of research in EBP and also the nature of knowledge for nursing practice in its many forms.

Parahoo, K (2014) *Nursing research: principles, process and issues* (3rd edn). London: Palgrave Macmillan.

Especially Chapters 1 and 2. These chapters explore the role of research in nursing practice and the nature of knowledge for nursing practice.

Useful websites

http://clinicalevidence.bmj.com/ceweb/index.html This is an interesting, very clinically orientated website that examines the evidence around a variety of medical conditions and is regularly updated.

www.casp-uk.net The home of the Critical Appraisal Skills Programme, an Oxford-based organisation concerned with improving the understanding of research evidence in health and social care.

www.cochrane.org The home of over 5000 systematic clinical evidence reviews.

www.evidence.nhs.uk This provides access to the latest clinical and non-clinical evidence for practice. Click on the 'A–Z of Topics' tab and select a clinical condition. Pay special attention to the 'Evidence Uncertainty' tab; here you will find numerous examples of areas of practice where the evidence remains questionable.

www.nice.org.uk This is the website for the National Institute for Health and Care Excellence where you might examine some of the criteria NICE uses in order to evaluate medications and interventions for clinical practice.

Chapter 2
Sources of knowledge for evidence-based care

Caroline Thomas

NMC Standards for Pre-registration Nursing Education

This chapter will address the following competencies:

Domain 1: Professional values

7. All nurses must be responsible and accountable for keeping their knowledge and skills up to date through continuing professional development. They must aim to improve their performance and enhance the safety and quality of care through evaluation, supervision and appraisal.

8. All nurses must practise independently, recognising the limits of their competence and knowledge. They must reflect on these limits and seek advice from, or refer to, other professionals where necessary.

9. All nurses must appreciate the value of evidence in practice, be able to understand and appraise research, apply relevant theory and research findings to their work, and identify areas for further investigation.

Domain 3: Nursing practice and decision-making

1. All nurses must use up-to-date knowledge and evidence to assess, plan, deliver and evaluate care, communicate findings, influence change and promote health and best practice. They must make person-centred, evidence-based judgements and decisions, in partnership with others involved in the care process, to ensure high-quality care. They must be able to recognise when the complexity of clinical decisions requires specialist knowledge and expertise, and consult or refer accordingly.

2. All nurses must possess a broad knowledge of the structure and functions of the human body, and other relevant knowledge from the life, behavioural and social sciences as applied to health, ill health, disability, ageing and death. They must have an in-depth knowledge of common physical and mental health problems and treatments in their own field of practice, including co-morbidity and physiological and psychological vulnerability.

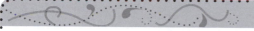

NMC Essential Skills Clusters

This chapter addresses the following ESCs:

Cluster: Care, compassion and communication
1(8). Demonstrates clinical confidence through sound knowledge, skills and understanding relevant to field.

Cluster: Organisational aspects of care
9 (14). Applies research-based evidence to practice.
15 (5). Recognises and addresses deficits in knowledge and skill in self and others and takes appropriate action.
16 (3). Bases decisions on evidence and uses experience to guide decision-making.

Chapter aims

After reading this chapter, you should be able to:

- describe the steps required to undertake a basic online search for evidence;
- identify key sources of appropriate evidence to inform nursing practice;
- demonstrate awareness of sources of health related policy in the United Kingdom;
- consider the reliability and trustworthiness of some key sources of evidence.

Introduction

Knowing how to search for, access and evaluate information is important for successful, high-quality, cost-effective practice in professional nursing and healthcare. Acquiring evidence can provide professionals with new insights into nursing practice and deepen their understanding of concepts central to nursing care. Possession of new insights can lead to improvements in care. Nurses need to develop a reflective approach to their practice, which includes finding out about the latest research and evaluating findings so the needs of patients and their families are responded to using the best available evidence. In addition, nurses need to know about the latest policies, standards and guidance determining their practice to ensure their practice is evidence-based. This requires understanding the process of searching for information and ways of appraising the authority and quality of information sources. The importance of assessing and evaluating sources of evidence is reflected in the Nursing and Midwifery Council *Standards for Pre-registration Nursing Education* (2010).

This chapter outlines basic search techniques that can be used to find evidence and offers guidance on ways of evaluating the credibility of information found. Defining and refining topics for consideration and following a series of stages to guide research are invaluable in making information searches efficient. This chapter also provides a variety of sources/resources that can be utilised to access reliable information for evidence-based practice.

To check learning, and make this chapter relevant to your current requirements, you are invited to follow the process and search for a topic, which would assist your assignment writing or deepen your understanding of an aspect of practice. You should bookmark the electronic sources you find or save your searches so that you can return to them in the future.

Scenario

Janice is 26, has completed an access course in health and social care and is starting an adult nursing programme at university. She is anxious to improve her library skills. She finds searching for information challenging and time-consuming. To improve her ability to research information she undertook a library workshop on 'developing skills for searching for information'.

The workshop content is detailed below.

The search process

Searching for quality information can be time-consuming. Therefore, knowing how to start a search and the steps to follow in undertaking a search can ensure time is used effectively. Having a search strategy can also prevent you being diverted to information only loosely connected to a topic. You have the option of searching manually or electronically, but electronic searches can increase the speed and ease of searching and are emphasised in this chapter.

There are three ways of gaining access to electronically stored evidence: free access, access paid for by institutions and access paid for by individuals. Specialist librarians for nursing, health and social care can provide valuable guidance on what sources of evidence are available and ways of undertaking searches.

A successful search strategy

A successful search entails collating information about the extent of relevant knowledge available. A clear search strategy begins with you defining the topic area, and following a series of interrelated steps:

Step 1: Definition of the research question, topic or area of enquiry

Step 2: Identification of a set of key words

Step 3: Refining or broadening the search

Step 4: Identification of appropriate sources of evidence

Step 5: Keeping a record of the search.

Step 1: Defining the research topic or question

Before starting your search, you need to determine what you need to find out about and the level of information required. In practice, this topic may stem from discussions with patients, a review of their notes or from discussions with colleagues or mentors. The topic may also relate to the pre-registration nursing standards or an assignment being assessed in a nursing programme or course.

> ### Example: You may wish to find out about the management of high blood pressure.
>
> *A range of factors can contribute to this, a range of treatments can be offered and different groups of patients can be affected. Deciding on the types of patient and whether you are interested in causes, treatments or all the aspects helps to limit your search and the time taken to do this.*

Step 2: Identification of key words

Identifying key words is essential for successful searches for evidence using indexes in books, electronic databases and search engines, such as Google Scholar. A good way to start is to break what you want to find out into a list of key words or concepts. This can take a few minutes if you are familiar with the topic. Be aware that different wording can be used to describe similar concepts relevant to the topic.

Example: *'Hypertension' means the same thing as 'high blood pressure'.* You can either record the key words in a list or as a mind map.

To broaden the list of key words, use of a dictionary or thesaurus can help; however, a general electronic thesaurus may not use a term in the same way as it is used in nursing or medicine.

Another useful source for key words is Wikipedia, a free online encyclopaedia. This should not, however, be used to provide references in academic assignments as experts in the field have not necessarily written or reviewed the information. The accuracy of the information can be questioned. Wikipedia is covered in the section on appropriate sources of information in this chapter.

Internet search engines, such as Google, Google Scholar or Google Chrome can reveal a range of items from the search but not all may be useful sources. By identifying key words you can reduce the number of hits to a manageable level.

A useful way of identifying key words in a topic is to use the PICO framework (Straus et al., 2010). This can be used to search for studies looking at the outcomes of interventions.

The search question = P + I + C + O

Where:

P = Problem

I = Intervention or treatment

C = Comparison (if needed)

O = Outcomes.

Useful questions for searches can also be devised using PICO. For example, questions may include:

- *What are the causes of high blood pressure in elderly people?*
- *How can high blood pressure in old people be reduced?*

Example: This list provides an example of the key words for researching hypertension in elderly patients:

- *Blood pressure*
- *Hypertension*
- *Old people/patient(s)*
- *Elderly people/patient(s)*
- *Geriatric(s)*
- *Care*
- *Regulation*
- *Symptoms*
- *Causes*
- *Guidelines*
- *Tests*
- *Risks*
- *Prevention*
- *Signs*

As you start searching you may be able to expand your list of key words and become more precise in the language used.

Step 3: Refining or extending the search

Once you have a set of words relevant to the search, you can look at ways in which key words relate to each other when using electronic sources such as databases, search engines and library catalogues.

Enclosing key words in quotation marks means that the words will be searched for as a phrase in the order that they are written.

Example: 'eating disorders' or 'high blood pressure'

When using Google Scholar as a search engine, a search for *'eating disorders'* produces fewer results than a search for *eating disorders*.

To explore the ways in which two or more key words or search terms relate to each other, you can use *Boolean operators*. These are the link words: AND, OR, NOT. They link key words in a search in a number of ways.

- **AND:** Linking key words with AND narrows a search. This allows you to link a patient group with a health condition, and symptoms with treatments.

Example: To find out about eating disorders in teenagers, the search would be: teenagers AND 'eating disorders'.

The search will only retrieve items that include all these words. A smaller number of results are found than when just searching for 'eating disorders'.

- **OR:** Using OR broadens a search and allows you to search for several different terms or synonyms used to specify the same thing. Authors may use different terms to describe what you are looking for.

Example: In looking for evidence on eating disorders in teenagers, OR can be used to describe the same subject: children OR teens OR adolescents OR young adults. Your search could be broadened and include more results by entering: 'eating disorders' AND children OR teenagers.

- **NOT:** Using NOT narrows a search by excluding key words. However, be cautious when using NOT to avoid accidental removal of too many results, including relevant results, from the search.

Example: A search using NOT anorexia excludes information specifically related to this condition. Your search would be: 'eating disorders' NOT anorexia AND teenagers. Alternatively, your search could be: 'eating disorders' AND teenagers NOT anorexia. There will be a slight variation in the number of results found depending on the word order.

This search reduces the number of hits or results quite significantly.

Another way of refining a search is to set a date limit on the search. This ensures that the most recent evidence or research is considered.

Step 4: Identification of appropriate sources of information

In order to analyse critically health related issues and evaluate practice, it is important to make use of authoritative, reliable sources of information. When tutors mark your assignments or mentors assess your explanation for the care suggested on placement, a key question asked is:

What evidence are you using to convince me that what you suggest/argue is reasonable?

Anecdotal evidence lacks robustness. It is considered unreliable and untrustworthy because it is based on hearsay. Other unsubstantiated forms of evidence also lack reliability and accuracy. There are lots of sources of information but those written by people not sufficiently qualified in the field may be inaccurate or flawed. It may also be poorly written or argued. Use of poor quality, unreliable or anecdotal evidence in a review of evidence or academic assignment can affect the credibility of the work. Some appropriate sources are explored in more depth in the 'Appropriate sources of information' section of this chapter.

Table 2.1: The various sources of information available to support professional practice	
Source of information	**Brief description**
Experts	For example: experienced and knowledgeable colleagues, specialists, mentors, patients, carers, social workers
Libraries and library catalogues	Sources and list of sources held by libraries: university, Trust and NHS evidence libraries
Journals and e-journals	Peer-reviewed articles and research reports
Books and e-books	Textbooks, manuals, electronic books
News and media	Media generated health information: newspaper articles, documentaries
Search engines	Electronic search mechanism providing access to key organisations, websites, publications
Key organisations: publications and websites	For example: publications and websites for National Institute for Health and Care Excellence and Department of Health
Web 2.0 technologies	Wikis such as Wikipedia, blogs, social networking sites
Bibliographic databases	Databases providing access to journals, research reports, systematic reviews, conference proceedings, theses

Authoritative sources can be found within university and Trust libraries where they have been recommended by professional staff. When joining a nursing programme it is important to spend time familiarising yourself with relevant sources of information as these can be used throughout your studies and professional career. Universities may offer workshops or online tutorials and notes on ways of accessing authoritative sources of information. It is important to learn, and where appropriate to seek help in learning, how to use the library catalogue and other electronic databases to access quality sources of information to keep abreast of developments in current practice.

Books, journals and conference papers published by professional organisations related to nursing or scholarly publishers are authoritative texts. Books and journals are peer reviewed by experts and editors in the field, who endorse the quality and credibility of the information. Submissions are required to meet established standards for publication.

Policy documents produced by government organisations or professional organisations in the field aimed at improving health and patient care are also reliable sources of information.

You may come across a range of views and perspectives on topics searched for. For evidence-based practice, you should present alternative perspectives, evaluate their usefulness in terms of the question or situation and present these together with the references to show where you found them.

Systematic reviews can communicate the methods, results and implications of large, complex quantitative studies about a clinical problem undertaken by other researchers simply. Systematic reviews tend to detail the studies included in the review.

Questions to aid evaluation of the trustworthiness of sources of information

There are a number of questions that you can ask about various sources of information, particularly websites, to check the extent of their reliability and authenticity before you use the information from them. These include:

Questions about the author:

- Who is the author of the information?
- Are the author's qualifications and/or professional credentials given to indicate that the author has the authority to write about the field?

Questions about the source/website:

- Who is funding or supporting the website/source?
- Is it an academic website produced by a university or other academic institution, a not-for-profit making organisation or a commercial company?
- Who is the intended audience for the website?

Questions about the age of the information:

- When was the information written? The date is often difficult to establish for some websites.
- When was the website created or last updated? Websites are unstable and are continuously updated.
- Is the website and/or the information still relevant?

Questions about objectivity (neutrality) and reliability of content:

- To what extent is the information given objective or unbiased? In being objective, the author should outline limitations of the information or provide more than one/a balanced perspective on an issue.
- To what extent does the evidence put forward relate to the claims/arguments being made?
- What is the quality of the writing like?
- Has the information been peer reviewed?

Once evidence has been obtained, it must be appraised for its integrity and applicability to the situation, clinical problem or patient so as to determine whether findings should be used for academic purposes or to inform practice. If there are any doubts about the information, it is best not to use it or to verify it elsewhere from a more reputable source. Such sources could be key organisations for healthcare, specified in the 'Appropriate sources of information' section of this chapter.

Authoritative, objective information with clear publication dates found on academic websites or those of key organisations related to nursing and bibliographic databases can generally be downloaded in a file such as in pdf form. Such sources should ensure that any research studies referred to were approved by an ethics committee and were conducted with the application of ethical principles to protect the interests of research participants.

The way of identifying the type of website accessed

When accessing websites, the type of organisation publishing the website can often be identified using the URL (Uniform Resource Locator). The URL consists of the domain name and several elements, for example the URL for Google is **www.google.co.uk**.

www.	This stands for 'world wide web'.
google.	This represents the sites, which have the rights to use this domain name.
co.	This is part of the domain name specifying the type of organisation (co. illustrates a corporate organisation/commercial company).
uk	This aspect specifies that it is a UK-based website. However, some websites with .uk may not be located in the UK.

Universities and colleges in the United Kingdom have ac.uk at the end of the URL. Local authorities and government organisations have gov.uk at the end of the URL and the NHS has nhs.uk at the end of the URL. As websites are unstable sources of information being continuously updated and developed, it is important to reference the date you accessed the information gained.

Step 5: Keeping a record of the search

Keeping a record of the search in terms of key words used, when and where they were used can enable you to find information again quickly or prevent you from losing track of valuable sources.

With electronic searches you may be able to save your search or print it out. Many bibliographic databases enable searches to be stored for future recall.

When you search online, your search is added to your *search history*. You can view this history following the appropriate onscreen links. You may also be able to edit your search history, save it and print it out so that you can use it again in the future without having to type in the website address or source.

It is possible to save many books and journals found in the electronic library databases. Librarians will be able to advise on this process.

Activity 2.1   *Reflection*

Janice found the above workshop content helped her to plan and conduct searches. She was also given a list of resources to access when writing her assignments.

Compare the existing ways you have searched for literature with the process described above. How might you narrow down your search for your chosen topic to ensure that it is manageable so that you access the most appropriate literature?

As this activity is based on your own observation, there is no outline answer at the end of the chapter.

Appropriate sources of information

Having established a strategy for organising a search on a relevant topic, you need to consider various appropriate sources of information that your searches may lead you to. These range from the opinions of experienced practitioners or specialist experts to research-based clinical guidelines or government health policy documents.

Activity 2.2   *Research and finding out*

Read the varied sources of information that can be accessed in the remainder of the chapter and allocate some time in the next couple of weeks to explore them. Note the type of resource accessed, such as a policy document, practice guidelines or research report. Identify what type of programme assignment or aspect of clinical practice each resource would provide evidence for.

As this activity is based on your own observation, there is no outline answer at the end of the chapter.

Experts

During your nursing career you will draw on a range of expertise to inform your practice: your personal experience as well as valuable insights or advice gained from patients, carers and colleagues. At the start of your nursing programme, mentors provide guidance, supervise and assess your practice. As your programme progresses you are expected to independently investigate topics, offer an evidence-based rationale for care delivered and question the practice of others. Through investigating a range of sources of evidence to support your practice, you will build up the knowledge base needed to support you throughout your professional career.

Libraries and library catalogues

University libraries

University libraries contain a range of journals and books that you can access on the shelves for nursing, which public libraries do not hold. An electronic *library catalogue* provides access to all the sources of information held by the library. This collection may include e-books, which are online versions of printed books, as well as electronic journals. When considering which sources to use, it is worthwhile consulting your programme/module handbook and bibliography for guidance.

You can search library catalogues by subject area or author. To locate a book on the shelves record the class mark. This is a series of letters and/or numbers. If the book is out on loan, you may find others with similar class marks on the shelves, covering the topic of interest. You can also search for newspapers, films and large print books.

Trust libraries

When on placement, you may utilise the Trust's library to aid your academic study and clinical practice. Trust librarians can provide information on your access rights to information, the sources available and ways of utilising the database to conduct searches. As a pre-registration nurse on a university programme, you can apply for free access to NHS Evidence, a library database providing access to a range of e-books, journals and practice guidelines.

Activity 2.3   *Critical thinking*

Consider the following scenario:

Gillian has started her child nursing programme, is confident in her IT and library skills, but was disappointed with her grade in her last academic assignment. The marker's comments suggested that she should make use of more creditable, professional sources of evidence to support her argument and not rely on information from Wikipedia and Google.

What sources of evidence would you recommend that Gillian could learn to access?

A possible outline answer can be found at the end of this chapter.

Journal articles

To check the relevance of a journal article identified by a search read the abstract, which is a brief summary of the article. It normally specifies the types of information being presented. This information can include randomised control trials, systematic reviews and small-scale studies on perspectives of care. This is a list of some journals publishing aspects related to nursing:

- *British Journal of Nursing* (Mark Allen Publishing)
- *International Journal of Nursing Studies*
- *Journal of Advanced Nursing*
- *Journal of Clinical Nursing*
- *Journal of Nursing Education*
- *Journal of Professional Nursing*
- *Nursing Standard* (Royal College of Nursing, Great Britain)
- *Nursing Times.*

Through looking at the reference list in relevant articles found you can broaden your search to include other relevant sources of information. It is worth finding out which e-journals for nursing your university library subscribes to.

You need to be aware that some journals have higher academic status than others in the field, as the standards for research reports are more rigorous. These journals tend to be cited more numerously by researchers in the field than others. The *International Journal of Nursing Studies* and *Journal of Advanced Nursing* are highly regarded sources of evidence-based information. The *Nursing Times* is a less rigorous source of evidence-based practice. It publishes professional and clinical news stories and comments from nurses in a 'magazine-style' format.

You may like to ask your health and social care librarian to show how to access the *impact factor* for nursing journals on the Web of Science electronic database. Journals are ranked according to their impact, i.e. the number of times they are cited in other publications and research. This provides an indication of their academic status in the field of nursing.

Google Books

Searching *Google Books* allows you access to extracts and information from a range of online books on a topic of your choice. Depending on the viewing permitted by publishers, you can obtain a summary of many books, browse the content or index pages and even read some parts or all of the books for free. You can also find out where to purchase or borrow a book you are interested in.

News and media

Newspapers and television provide information on healthcare for the public, and up-to-date news items related to issues concerning health and social care provision. Browsing the health pages of newspapers, news programmes and documentaries can provide insights into patient perspectives on healthcare and the findings of reviews of standards of care within Trusts. Articles and news stories can be subject to bias so the information gathered should be used as a stimulus for further investigation into the claims made using additional credible sources of evidence and not be used as a sole justification to alter practice.

Current news items and advice about health can be accessed using websites of some key organisations, news channels and newspapers. Examples include:

- BBC News: **www.bbc.co.uk/news/health**
- The Guardian: **www.theguardian.com/society/health**

Search engines

Many search engines have been designed to help find information on the web. These include: *Ask, Bing, Exalead, Google, Google Chrome and Google Scholar. Google Scholar* specifically focuses on enabling searches for scholarly literature (**http://scholar.google.co.uk**):

> *From one place, you can search across many disciplines and sources: articles, theses, books, abstracts and court opinions, from academic publishers, professional societies, online repositories, universities and other web sites. Google Scholar helps you find relevant work across the world of scholarly research.*

Google Scholar offers online advice on searching. It allows you to use key words and Boolean operators covered in this chapter to search for evidence and has an advanced search facility.

Key organisations: websites and publications

You can access a range of reliable, credible evidence from the websites of key organisations covered in the table below. Understanding the political context governing care in the UK is important as this has an impact on practice. The Department of Health database is one of the most important sources for this.

Web 2.0 technologies

Web 2.0 technologies are increasingly becoming a popular means of collecting research data and sharing research findings. These sources can include social networking sites such as Facebook

Table 2.2: Key health organisations, websites and the information available

Key organisation	Website	Useful sources of information
Department of Health (DH)	**www.gov.uk/ government/ organisations/ department-of-health**	The DH publishes a range of information covering policy announcements, policy consultations and standards relevant to nursing, midwifery and healthcare in the UK.
		A range of policies, publications on healthcare and national news items related to health can be accessed using the website. Up-to-date statistics on a range of topics such as specific health conditions, births and patient experience are also available.
		There is a link to the NHS for information on the constitution and role of the National Health Service.
		Details of the ministers at the DH are also given.
National Institute for Health and Care Excellence (NICE)	**www.nice.org.uk**	NICE is an independent organisation, providing current evidence-based information for health, public health and social care.
		NICE develops quality standards and guidelines, designed to improve particular areas of health in conjunction with health and social care professionals, their partners and service users. The standards are reviewed annually and can be accessed online.
		'Local practice collection', accessible via the website, provides examples of the use of NICE guidance and standards to improve health.
		The online 'evidence search' allows access to research on a range of topics, links to the Cochrane Library and access to e-books and e-journals using OpenAthens account held with your university library.
		NICE also provides access to the NHS evidence database.
NHS England NHS Scotland NHS Wales Health and Social Care Services in Northern Ireland	**www.england. nhs.uk www. healthscotland. com www.wales.nhs. uk http://online. hscni.net**	NHS England leads the National Health Service (NHS) in England. It establishes the priorities and direction of the NHS, and encourages and informs the national debate to improve health and care.
		The website provides access to information on patient engagement in healthcare, structure of the healthcare system, the vision for the future and information about health issues.

(Continued)

Table 2.2: (Continued)

Key organisation	Website	Useful sources of information
		Websites also exist detailing the structure and nature of healthcare provision in Wales, Scotland and Northern Ireland.
Nursing and Midwifery Council (NMC)	**www.nmc.org.uk**	The NMC is a statutory body regulating the nursing and midwifery profession so as to protect the public.
		The website provides access to the Code for nurses and midwives: the professional standards that nurses and midwives must uphold in order to be registered to practise in the UK.
		The website provides useful information in the context of care. Understanding this can aid understanding of the credibility and usefulness of evidence for practice.
		Employers can use the website to check the registration status of employees.
Royal College of Nursing (RCN)	**www.rcn.org.uk**	The RCN is a membership organisation for registered nurses, midwives, healthcare assistants and nursing students. It is a professional body, working on nursing standards, education and practice, and a trade union. It has one of the largest nursing libraries in Europe. Its database enables access to a large collection of e-books and e-journals. It produces a range of quality publications.
		The RCN website provides advice on professional development. A section is devoted to students with resources, events and opportunities to support your studies and search for your first job.
World Health Organization (WHO)	**www.who.int/ about/en**	The WHO directs and coordinates international health within the United Nations' system.
		The website provides details of the work of the WHO, its publications, classification of diseases and the tackling of current international health priorities.

and Twitter. They also include blogs, wikis such as Wikipedia, podcasts and video-sharing sites such as YouTube. Many journals are now promoted on Twitter (**www.twitter.com**). Twitter is a way of communicating information through Tweets using a limited number of characters.

Using social media technologies, users can interact, share content and have conversations. Networks can be created between similar professionals enabling the sharing of expertise in the field.

Blogs can be web-based conversations or diaries, which exist around a theme. Blogs may hold a series of opinions or comments on news items, policies and issues related to health. Patients may provide narratives of their health conditions, comment on their experiences of care and suggest improvements for other people. Contributors are invited to write postings, which vary in terms of length and quality. Nurses and pre-registration nurses are invited to share experiences and discuss articles on the evidence-based nursing blog. For further information access: **http://blogs. bmj.com/ebn/ebn-twitter-journal-club**.

The King's Fund, an independent charity organisation involved in promoting an understanding of the health and social care system, provides access to a blog on patient experiences and views of care in the UK: **www.kingsfund.org.uk/blog**.

Caution is needed when making reference to social media sites or blogs in academic work. It is not easy to determine the authority of the information. Whilst unique perspectives of individuals can be of value, as long as they are authentic, they can also be biased. Consequently findings should not be used to generalise the viewpoints described as representative of the general population. However, gaining an insight into a range of different patient perspectives can be helpful in terms of making you more sensitive to the varying needs of patients with specific conditions.

Wikipedia

Wikipedia is a free online encyclopaedia and provides a good starting point for finding out about a topic and key words for searches. However, any registered user can alter an article so the accuracy and authenticity of the information can be questioned. Articles are continuously being rewritten. References to each entry or topic are often given at the end and can be checked and compared with other reputable sources.

Bibliographic databases

University libraries subscribe to bibliographic databases. These give nurses access through a user name and password to a wealth of published literature, including articles, conference proceedings, research reports, newspaper articles, theses or systematic reviews. Many have menus with onscreen instructions making the retrieval of evidence straightforward. Information is often presented as a reference and a summary of the text. Librarians are able to advise on access rights and use of these.

Depending on your access rights, you may be able to download the full text of some articles. If you are unable to retrieve an article, make a record of the reference so you can enquire about obtaining this through the interlibrary loan system.

Examples of useful subject specific databases

When using bibliographic databases, those relevant to nursing will be most useful to you. These include CINAHL (Cumulative Index to Nursing and Allied Health Literature), British Nursing Index, PsycINFO (which covers aspects related to psychology) and Allied and Complementary

Medicine. These all hold references on nursing related studies. These may be accessible via the internet or your university library.

Table 2.3: Subject specific bibliographic databases relevant to nurses		
British Nursing Index	**www.proquest. com/products-services/bni.html**	• UK nursing and midwifery database compiled by professional librarians • Covers over 400 UK journals and other English language titles, including international nursing and midwifery journals, as well as selective content from medical, allied health and management titles • Updated monthly (for core UK nursing and midwifery)
Cumulative Index to Nursing and Allied Health Literature CINAHL	**https://health. ebsco.com/ products/the-cinahl-database**	• Provides access to nursing and allied health literature including nursing journals, conference proceedings and publications from the National League for Nursing, and the American Nurses' Association • Literature covers a range of topics such as nursing, biomedicine, health sciences, complementary medicine and consumer health • Provides access to healthcare books, nursing dissertations, selected conference proceedings, standards of practice, audiovisuals and book chapters
MEDLINE	**https://health. ebsco.com/ products/medline**	• Created by US National Library of Medicine • Contains citations and abstracts for biomedical and health journals • Used by healthcare professionals, nurses, clinicians and researchers engaged in care, public health and health policy development
The Cochrane Library	**www.cochrane library.com/about/ about-the-cochrane-library.html** **www.cochrane library.com/ cochrane-database-of-systematic-reviews/index.html**	• Produces up-to-date research evidence • Has a number of databases • Cochrane Database of Systematic Reviews (CDSR) is a leading database for healthcare, publishing systematic reviews of randomised controlled trials, editorials and the protocols for Cochrane Reviews • You can search by topic or each Cochrane Review Group (CGG), which takes responsibility for a specific area of healthcare or policy

Joanna Briggs Institute of Systematic Reviews and Implementation reports	**http://joannabriggs library.org/index. php/jbisrir**	• A refereed online journal • Publishes systematic review protocols and systematic reviews of healthcare research following the JBI methodology undertaken by the Joanna Briggs Institute, its international collaborating centres and groups
PsycINFO	**www.apa.org/ pubs/databases/ psycinfo/**	• PsycINFO is a specialist database for locating scholarly research findings in psychology and related fields • Contains access to journals, books and reports
Applied Social Sciences Index and Abstracts (ASSIA)	**www.proquest. com/products-services/ASSIA-Applied-Social-Sciences-Index-and-Abstracts.html**	• Useful database for community nursing, containing information on a topic that has a social as well as a medical/nursing focus, such as domestic violence

Activity 2.4

Select a health related topic you wish to learn about (e.g. consider the ways of preventing the onset of common colds). Conduct a search using the electronic library catalogue or a search engine of your choice to find three relevant journal articles.

Read the title and abstract for each article. Note the dates of publication. Determine whether they look relevant. Access the full text version and look for information, which tells you whether the author is a credible authority on the subject. How detailed is the content? Are references used to support any claims made?

As this is based on your own observation, there is no outline answer at the end of the chapter.

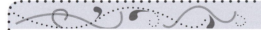

Chapter summary

This chapter has outlined the following:

• A variety of appropriate sources, from within and outside the field of nursing, that can be used to assist evidence-based practice.
• The importance of planning a search strategy, making notes and following a simple process for conducting searches for evidence using key words and Boolean operators.
• Questions that can be used to help evaluate the quality and authority of sources of evidence.

continued ...

- The need to familiarise yourself with sources of information that are most relevant so that these can be revisited regularly to help you keep up to date with developments in practice.
- The importance of seeking support from subject specialist librarians on sources of information and searches.

Clearly, the better informed you are as a nurse the more likely it is that you will provide high standards of care and achieve successful outcomes for your patients. It is hoped that this chapter encourages you to seek out the information you need to better understand how to care for your patients and prepare for your written assessments.

Activity: Brief outline answer

Activity 2.3: Critical thinking (page 34)

Gillian may find it helpful to use Google Scholar to access more academic material to use in her assignments. She could also enquire about tutorials or workshops to assist her in the use of the library catalogue.

She will need to master ways of accessing bibliographic databases so that she can access full-text journal articles.

She could access more professional sources of information through using websites such as NICE and the Royal College of Nursing. Websites such as the Department of Health will help her develop an understanding of the influence policy has on practice.

Further reading

Gerrish, K and Lathlean, J (eds) (2015) *The research process in nursing* (7th edn). Chichester: John Wiley & Sons.

Moule, P and Goodman, M (2014) *Nursing research: an introduction* (2nd edn). London: Sage.

Schmidt, NA and Brown, JM (eds) (2015) *Evidence-based practice for nurses: appraisal and application* (3rd edn). Burlington, USA: Jones & Bartlett.

Useful websites

www.evidence.nhs.uk National Health Service (NHS) Evidence. This provides access to a range of resources, including the British National Formulary (BNF), which illustrates which drugs are used to treat conditions occurring in different parts of the body.

www.gov.uk/government/organisations/department-of-health Department of Health website. This provides access to national health policy information.

www.kingsfund.org.uk King's Fund website.

www.nice.org.uk National Institute for Health and Care Excellence website.

www.nmc.org.uk Nursing and Midwifery Council (NMC) website.

www.ons.gov.uk Office for National Statistics website. Provides statistical data on diseases and treatments that can be used when explaining the context to a health topic. An example includes the mortality rates for different conditions.

www.rcn.org.uk Royal College of Nursing (RCN).

Chapter 3
Critiquing research: the generic elements

Peter Ellis

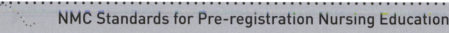

NMC Standards for Pre-registration Nursing Education

This chapter will address the following competencies:

Domain 3: Nursing practice and decision-making
1. All nurses must use up-to-date knowledge and evidence to assess, plan, deliver and evaluate care, communicate findings, influence change and promote health and best practice. They must make person-centred, evidence-based judgements and decisions, in partnership with others involved in the care process, to ensure high-quality care.
10. All nurses must evaluate their care to improve clinical decision-making, quality and outcomes, using a range of methods, amending the plan of care, where necessary, and communicating changes to others.

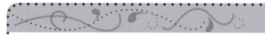

NMC Essential Skills Clusters

This chapter will address the following ESCs:

Cluster: Care, compassion and communication
1. As partners in the care process, people can trust a newly registered graduate nurse to provide collaborative care based on the highest standards, knowledge and competence.

Cluster: Organisational aspects of care
12. People can trust the newly registered graduate nurse to respond to their feedback and a wide range of other sources to learn, develop and improve services.

Chapter aims

After reading this chapter, you will be able to:

*   demonstrate awareness of the need for critical reviewing of research in health and social care;

- describe the type of questions that can be applied to all research papers during the critiquing process;
- demonstrate awareness of the systematic nature of the process of research critiquing;
- understand the ethical considerations that need to be taken into account when evaluating health and social care research.

Introduction

In this book we have established that it is important for nurses who wish to be truly evidence-based to be critical and analytical in their approach to the identification, reading and potential adoption into their practice of various sources of evidence. We have already indicated that an understanding of research **methodologies**, **methods** and analysis is useful in establishing the worth of **empirical** literature to inform evidence-based nursing practice.

The opportunities for every nurse to engage in clinical research are limited, and there are good reasons why this should be the case. Prime among these is the potential for overwhelming both practice and patients with requests to participate in research, thereby detracting from the delivery of good quality clinical care. Rather, the challenge is for nurses to engage with research as an important source of evidence to guide and inform practice. One practical mechanism for doing this is via a work-based or university journal club that might meet to identify, critique and discuss the adoption of new research findings.

Renewal of registration and revalidation according to the Code Paragraph 22 (NMC, 2015) requires nurses to: *keep your knowledge and skills up to date, taking part in appropriate and regular learning and professional development activities that aim to maintain and develop your competence and improve your performance.* Clearly therefore one of the requirements for revalidation of nurses is that they engage in continuing professional development and that they maintain a record of reflection; it would therefore be a good habit for nursing students to develop and registered nurses to continue with (Ellis and Abbott, 2015).

Regardless of whether all nurses are able to undertake research, they should have at least a basic understanding of how research is undertaken, and what constitutes good-quality research fit to inform their practice. Being able to judge the quality of a piece of research and its applicability to our individual clinical settings and client groups is essential if we are to use it to inform what we do in a meaningful way. So as well as being able to critique research, nurses need to understand whether the research might be useful in informing practice where they work.

It is beyond the scope of this book to look in detail at the design and execution of the various forms of research used to inform nursing practice. For a detailed look at the design and undertaking of research studies in nursing practice, or to help you with a critique of a piece of research, see *Understanding Research for Nursing Students* (also in this series – other sources you may wish to use are identified at the end of this chapter).

Because there is a need to understand some general areas for critique as well as how to critique the specifics of the two main approaches to research, qualitative and quantitative methodologies, this part of the book is split into two chapters. The first, this chapter, the generic section, deals with critiquing elements of published research that apply to *all* research papers of whatever methodology. This includes the titles, authors, choice of research **paradigm** and the discussion and conclusions sections of the paper as well as some consideration of the ethical questions that might be asked of a published study. The next chapter (Chapter 4) will focus on specific questions to be asked of qualitative and quantitative research. Areas for critique within Chapter 4 include methodological choice (design), sampling, data-collection methods and analysis of the data.

Within both chapters there are some brief descriptions and critiques of elements of various research papers. Most of these papers are readily available via university or hospital based journal subscriptions both online and on paper. Where possible, it would help your understanding of the process of research critiquing to read some of these papers in full, although this is not absolutely necessary. Chapter 2 will help you to work out how to access these papers using electronic database searches – the details of which are explored in the book *Information Skills for Nursing Students*, also in this series.

As well as the guidance contained within these chapters there is a comprehensive critiquing framework in the Appendix that can be applied to most research. This framework is in three sections: the first applies to all research, as does this chapter; the second has additional questions that apply to qualitative research (see Chapter 4); and the third has additional questions that relate to quantitative research (also in Chapter 4). You might find it useful to read both chapters while simultaneously referring to the questions contained in this framework. Because the critiquing of research is a dynamic process where a number of judgement calls need to be made, the contents of the chapters and the questions within the framework do not exactly mirror each other.

It is important to establish right from the start that critiquing in this sense is seen not merely as an activity that is used to identify weaknesses within a study, but also as an activity that seeks to establish a study's strengths and therefore the degree of faith that can be placed in its findings. So, as in the rest of the book, the critical activities are seen not merely as a means to establish weakness but also as a means of identifying good-quality evidence that may subsequently be useful in the advancement of practice. Clearly, this cannot be achieved if the sole intention of the activity is to identify and discard weak research.

The format of the presentation of this and the following chapter is intended not only to help you ask the right question of the different areas of the research papers you read but also to provide you with what you might be looking for in the way of a positive answer to the question posed. The questions and guidance in these two chapters, along with the framework in the Appendix, can be used to provide a map for undertaking a critique of a research paper in a meaningful and straightforward manner.

While much of what you will need to ask and the sort of answers that you will be looking for is contained within these chapters and the Appendix, this does not negate the need for some further reading around the methodologies and methods of the papers you may be using these chapters to help critically analyse.

If you are undertaking a critique as part of some course work, you should also refer to the assignment guidelines and ensure that you only appraise the elements of the research you are asked to critique.

Undertaking the critique

There is no single right way to approach undertaking a critique of a piece of research. There are, however, some strategies that will make the process easier for the novice to undertake and that can provide structure to the process.

Lobiondo-Wood and Haber (2013) suggest the following strategy:

- Skim read the paper to get a feel for the overall approach of the research.

- Read the paper in depth, making sure you understand each element.

- Break the study down into its component parts.

- Think about the study as a whole and consider its message.

Certainly, these are useful strategies. Highlighting important areas of the text is also useful as is drawing a simple flow diagram of the research, including the question, methodology, sample, methods, analysis, results and key discussion points, which makes referring back to the paper much easier to do and aids in the critiquing process (see Figure 3.1). A short overview of each piece of research is very helpful where you are considering critiquing a number of research papers, as you might in a review, for example.

A much briefer flow diagram of such research can prove useful for gaining an overview of a single piece of research and for comparing the processes with a number of different research studies. In fact, the Consolidated Standards of Reporting Trials (CONSORT) group, who are concerned with improving the reporting of clinical trials, have created a flow diagram for this very purpose, which demonstrates how data can be downsized into manageable chunks for the purposes of review. Clearly, this template applies only to clinical trials and shows participant movement through a trial, but the idea can be adapted to suit all research methodologies and further notes can be added as required.

Activity 3.1   *Research and finding out*

Visit the CONSORT website at **www.consort-statement.org/consort-statement/flow-diagram0/** and download a copy of the flow diagram. Take some time to look over the way in which it is presented and consider how you might use and adapt it for yourself.

As this activity is based on your own observations, there is no outline answer at the end of the chapter.

A further useful (and often overlooked) part of the process of an academic critique is the use of research resources to inform the process. This involves using books about research to highlight the processes a research study might undertake in the ideal world. What actually happened in the study you are reviewing is then compared to these processes as part of your critique.

Of course, it is often the case that you will understand different sections in certain books better than in others, so use more than one textbook against which to compare the research that you are reading.

Furze, G, Cox, H, Morton, V, Chuang, L-H, Lewin, RJP, Nelson, P, Carty, R, Norris, H, Patel, N and Elton, P (2012) Randomized controlled trial of a lay-facilitated angina management programme. *Journal of Advanced Nursing*, 68(10): 2267–79.

Aims: To establish the relative effectiveness and comparative costs associated with a home-based, lay-facilitated Angina Management Programme when compared to routine advice and education from a specialist nurse.

Methodology: Randomised controlled trial.

Sample: Adult patients with angina in rapid-access chest pain clinic at a district general hospital; excluding: need for urgent revascularisation, exercise-induced arrhythmias, loss of systolic BP greater than 20 mmHg during exercise stress testing, increasing number and duration of attacks of angina; a score of 4 on the Canadian Angina Class or the New York Heart Association classification of heart failure; life-threatening co-morbidities; certain psychiatric problems. 142 recruited (sample size calculation suggests 158).

Methods: Intervention group: Angina Plan (education about angina, exercise, stress management referral for smoking cessation) delivered and monitored by trained lay persons. Control group: seen by specialist nurse in clinic and given usual advice.

Analysis: Intention to treat analysis (includes withdrawals to reflect true life). Regression modelling used. Number of angina episodes over six months plus blood pressure, cholesterol, body mass index, waist/hip ratio, Seattle Angina Questionnaire and Hospital Anxiety and Depression Scales. Cost-effectiveness assessed using Quality Adjusted Life Years.

Results: No important difference in frequency of angina at six months. Positive differences for intervention group, at three months for anxiety, understanding and exercise; and at six months for anxiety, depression and understanding. The intervention was considered cost-effective.

Discussion: Some outcomes are better within the Angina Plan delivered by lay persons than standard advice presented in the clinic by a specialist nurse.

Figure 3.1: Example overview of a randomised controlled trial

Theory

When undertaking an assignment as part of a course or module of study, it is usual to follow certain academic conventions. The need to follow these conventions is no different when undertaking a critique. The usual strategy when approaching this sort of work is to define your terms (explain what a technical word means); reference the definition (to an academic text such as a research textbook); and apply the definition to the critique you are undertaking. There is then a higher probability that you understand the new terminology and that the marker understands what it is you are trying to say and is sure that you understand what it is you are saying; this process of define, reference and apply is a good tool for all forms of academic work.

Many textbooks and websites about research and evidence-based practice contain frameworks that can be used to guide the process of critiquing a research paper (see the Further reading section at the end of the chapter). They point the reader in the direction of the correct questions to ask at the different stages of the review; in general, they are best used in conjunction with at least one research textbook. It is important to ascertain what types of research the frameworks are written in relation to, as some are generic (that is, they apply to all methodologies) while others are specific to either the **qualitative** or **quantitative paradigms**, and yet others relate only to individual specific methodologies. The critiquing framework presented in the Appendix is both generic (it can be used to ask questions of all research methodologies) and specific (it contains paradigm-specific elements).

Concept summary: quantitative and qualitative research

Quantitative research is associated with scientific enquiry that views the world in a measurable, 'provable' manner. 'Quantitative' refers to the fact that findings are countable or can be presented in numbers, tables and graphs. Quantitative research is concerned with proof, with cause and effect, and with demonstrating associations. Quantitative research often starts with a **hypothesis**, an idea to be tested using scientific methods.

Qualitative research is associated with the social sciences and 'people-centred' enquiry. 'Qualitative' refers to looking at the world from the point of view of what people feel, think, understand and believe – things that cannot easily be measured or counted. It is not so concerned with proof as with describing and understanding experiences from the viewpoint of people who have had, or are having, the experience in question. Qualitative research starts with a question and may be used to generate a hypothesis, but does not start with one.

Generic questions

There are some questions that apply to all the research papers that you might read. These generic questions relate to some of the core decisions about the general approach to the research being undertaken, how ethically the research has been undertaken and, to a lesser extent, the title of the paper and the credentials of the authors. There are some common pitfalls and assumptions that students make when critiquing research that will be identified below, and some ideas about how to overcome these and establish the quality of the critique being undertaken.

This notion of the quality of the critique is in many respects as important as the notion of the quality of the research paper. If the idea of learning to prepare, and indeed undertaking, a research critique is to provide evidence to inform clinical practice, then the process by which this is achieved must also be robust. Clearly, this is also important for the student who is seeking to gain a good mark for a piece of course work as well!

Title

Many critiquing frameworks require the user to make decisions about the quality of some issues relating to the title of the paper being critiqued. Certainly, it is very frustrating to find that the content of a paper bears no resemblance to what appears in the title. There can also be an issue with being able to identify from a paper's title that it is a research paper rather than a review or an opinion piece.

The truth of the matter is that more often than not the authors of journal papers have limited input into the title their paper is given. The journal staff sometimes choose the title of the paper as a means of attracting potential readers to both the individual article and the journal.

Activity 3.2   *Reflection*

How might you know that you are reading a journal paper which is original research rather than some other type of publication such as a review or opinion paper?

An outline answer is provided at the end of the chapter.

Clearly, if you are required to critique elements of a research paper such as the title as part of some course work, then you must; ordinarily, however, it is not considered an important element of the critiquing process. As a general rule, a good title will identify the characteristics of the participants (e.g. people with diabetes), the nature of the research questions (e.g. quality of life) and the methodological approach used (e.g. **phenomenology**). Some titles may also include some message about the key findings of the research, although this is not always possible.

Author credentials

In essence, the author credentials are not as important as the quality of the research itself as all researchers have to start with a first paper and therefore limited publishing credentials (Coughlan et al., 2007). Checking the authors' credentials requires understanding of at least one of three main areas: their qualifications, their current and past work roles and their publication history.

It may be preferable for someone undertaking nursing research to have a nursing background and this may be established within the paper. Many journals do not publish authors' qualifications, however, so this is not always easily ascertained. It would therefore not be possible to critique credibility from this angle.

The author's role(s) can give a reasonable insight into what experience they have of the topic at hand – many journals publish this. Although we said that it may be preferable for nursing research to be undertaken by nurses, this certainly does not exclude research undertaken by people with other professional or academic backgrounds. Much of the knowledge base for nursing has been gained from other professional and academic disciplines, so it is common for individuals other than nurses to contribute to or undertake research that is applicable to nursing.

The third strategy that can be applied to establishing the author's credentials is to look at their publication history. This can often be achieved by finding their profile(s) (where these exist) – for example, on a university website – and where these are not available, by doing an author search on a bibliographic database to identify papers they have published on the topic of interest. A note of caution: sometimes the author with the research expertise is not the first author; for example, when a lecturer publishes work together with a research student, it may be necessary to search for more than just the first author.

The choice of research paradigm

The choice of research paradigm will depend on the type of question – or questions – that a piece of research is setting out to answer (Polit and Beck, 2013). Essentially, in health and social care (including nursing) research there are two distinct research paradigms. These paradigms represent two distinct, but not entirely separate, philosophical ways of viewing the world and asking questions. You may be familiar with the terms for these philosophical approaches: the qualitative paradigm and the quantitative paradigm (see Concept summary on pp51–2).

Given the differences between quantitative and qualitative paradigms, it is apparent that the approach to answering a question arising from nursing practice will depend on the nature of the question. Questions that focus on how people experience their world, what their attitudes are and how they perceive things will sit within the qualitative paradigm and will require that qualitative methodologies and methods are used to investigate them, while questions about cause and effect and things that can be enumerated will require a quantitative research approach. The two world views are not interchangeable in terms of asking specific research questions; however, many authors use methods for research data collection which are questionable given the question they are posing. For example it is quite common to see questionnaires used to collect qualitative data, but as we shall see the value of questionnaires (essentially a quantitative method) in qualitative research is itself questionable.

> **Concept summary: triangulation**
>
> Given the differences in approach to asking and answering questions, it would seem logical to expect to see research using either a qualitative or a quantitative approach to answering questions. While this is often the case, some research employs mixed methodologies and methods in order to look at a research question from more than one angle – this is called **triangulation**.
>
> *(Continued)*

(Continued)

This triangulation of methodologies and methods allows the researchers not only to ask questions about *what* happens under which circumstances and *how* it happens (as in quantitative research) but also to explore *why* people behave as they do or have the beliefs and opinions that they express (as in qualitative research). For example, *quantitatively* it can be demonstrated that a diet that is high in saturated fats is bad for health. In order to address individuals' eating behaviours, however, it is first necessary to understand, using *qualitative* methods, why people make the lifestyle choices they do.

The background/introduction/literature review, which is at the start of all good research papers, will help establish the credentials of the study as a qualitative or quantitative study (Moule, 2015). A good introduction will explore the state of the literature about the topic of interest and will establish what important older (but recent) research has shown about it.

Essentially, it is usual for the argument put forward in the introduction to the paper to lead the reader to the point where they can appreciate the sorts of questions that need answering about the topic of the research.

It is these questions posed in the introduction that will frame the research as either quantitative or qualitative.

Example critique: choice of paradigm

Virdee et al. (2015) used a qualitative research methodology in their study of people's views of using a polypill (a pill with multiple active ingredients to treat more than one disease, e.g. to lower blood pressure, lower cholesterol and act as a blood thinner) for the management of cardiovascular risk. Since this study is concerned with the views of the participants and not measuring the efficacy of the polypill, then a qualitative approach makes sense.

Questions posed in quantitative research are about proof, about cause and effect, and demonstrating potential associations between **variables**. Quantitative research often starts with a hypothesis, which is essentially an idea that is tested using established scientific methods. Hypotheses are often presented as a **null hypothesis** (or the opposite of what the researcher actually expects to find) in order to aid statistical analysis, which will disprove the null hypothesis, or prove the hypothesis, if you like.

Example of a quantitative research hypothesis

In their study of student nurses to compare face-to-face and computer-aided learning (CAL) about handwashing, Bloomfield et al. (2010, p289) posed three null hypotheses:

1. *There would be no difference between the knowledge test scores of nursing students taught the theory of handwashing using CAL when compared with those taught using conventional methods.*
2. *There would be no difference in the handwashing skill performance scores of nursing students taught using CAL when compared with those taught using conventional methods.*
3. *There would be no difference in the retention of handwashing knowledge and skills in nursing students taught handwashing using CAL when compared with those taught by conventional methods.*

These hypotheses appear to reflect the purpose of this form of enquiry, which is to understand whether computer-aided learning can assist the understanding of handwashing over three domains of measurement: knowledge, practice and retention of knowledge.

Qualitative questions seek answers about things that cannot easily be measured or counted. They are more concerned with understanding experiences, opinions and beliefs. Qualitative research starts with a question, an aim or a general statement about something that needs exploring; it does not start with a hypothesis but may be used to generate one.

Example of a qualitative research aim

In their qualitative study of the factors which stop suicide attempts in men, Player et al. (2015) pose the aim of their study as examining factors assisting, complicating or inhibiting interventions for men at risk, as well as outlining the roles of family, friends and others in male suicide prevention. Given that qualitative research is **inductive**, this aim, which contains no reference to the findings of the study and does not pose a hypothesis, appears to be appropriate to this research enquiry.

Critiquing the choice of paradigm, therefore, requires that you know what the two research paradigms are used to investigate and the sorts of questions they can answer. On some occasions it appears evident from the introduction that the answers to the important questions being asked lie in more than one paradigm, and that the researcher may be under-investigating the topic by failing to use a triangulated methodology.

Ethics

Ethics should permeate the whole research process. Good research is ethical research, but sadly not all ethical research is good research. Certainly, it is possible to undertake research that is both ethical and of a high standard, and in many respects producing research ethically adds to the quality of the research process.

When critiquing research from an ethical point of view, there are many questions that can and should be asked. Many students look for some statement that the research has been given ethical clearance, and many regard this as showing that the research is therefore ethically sound. There are two problems with adopting this stance: the first is that not all papers make this statement (Jolley, 2010); and the second is that even with ethical clearance, there may still be questions about the conduct of the research that need to be answered.

Concept summary: critiquing journal papers

One note of caution for the novice at critiquing is that many journals only accept papers that can demonstrate ethical clearance at the point of submission. In such journals the individual papers will not state that they received ethical clearance. It is worth checking either inside the journal itself or on the journal website where they carry 'information for authors' for a statement about the requirements for demonstrating ethical clearance for all research papers prior to acceptance – not only will this inform your critique but it is likely to impress your marker too.

Critiquing the ethical credentials of a paper starts with asking questions about whether the research was necessary or whether the existing research, which is covered in the background to the paper, suggests it is not. Undertaking research that is unnecessary is ethically questionable because of the use of resources, including people's time and energy. One also has to consider the emotional investment people make in the research process where they hope the research they are participating in may be of benefit to them or to other people in the future; it is therefore unethical to ask people to participate in research which has previously been proven to be futile or of general benefit; in the latter case people should just be offered the **gold standard** care.

Gaining **consent** is an ethical cornerstone of any research. Gaining true and valid consent is especially challenging in health and social care research because the participants have the potential to be vulnerable. This vulnerability may result from the participants being ill, elderly or in a dependent relationship with the researcher (who may also be their nurse or otherwise involved in their care). Gaining true consent requires the researcher to demonstrate that the participants' agreement to participate has been free from any coercion, either real or potential (Beauchamp and Childress, 2013).

Coupled with the issue of potential coercion are questions about the ability of the individuals to make a choice about whether to take part in a study or not. This freedom of choice is best illustrated in those studies that report that the participants know that they do not have to take part in the study and that they are aware that they can withdraw at any stage without compromising their usual care – although where this is not stated it is hard to know if this principle has been observed.

Consent also requires that the potential participants have the **capacity** (mental ability) to make the choice to participate or not. If there is any doubt about capacity, it is desirable that other sources of consent are sought, for instance from spouses, parents or other guardians (this is sometimes referred to as **assent**). In studies where there are obvious questions about the capacity of the participants to consent to taking part, it is desirable that the researchers make some statement about ethically managing this.

Example critique: consent

In their study into the use of assistive technology in people with dementia, Gibson et al. (2015) only included people in the study if they had enough capacity to be able to provide 'formal consent'. This demonstrates that Gibson et al. are showing respect for persons by not exploiting people who are incapable of providing consent; although given that the main method used for data collection was interviews, there are also practical reasons as to why the participants with dementia need the capability to communicate.

Other fundamental questions to be asked of the ethics of a paper include: Do they protect the **confidentiality** and **anonymity** of those involved? Do they appear to have done more good than harm? Did the study answer the question as set and were the resources used in the study used to good effect?

Activity 3.3   *Reflection*

Review what the Code says about consent and confidentiality. Reflect on what this means for undertaking nursing research.

As this activity is based on your own reflection, there is no outline answer at the end of the chapter.

All of these ethical questions can be asked in the critique, especially where the paper does not explicitly state whether the researchers have addressed them. A good study will not only state what ethical questions there are, but also suggest how these might have been addressed. For example, a good paper will make it clear that the researchers dealt with any upset caused by making counselling and support available.

There are many sources of questions about the ethics of research and how these should apply to the conduct of research in human subjects. Some general ethical principles that guide this questioning have already been identified, but Beauchamp and Childress (2013) identify four important ethical principles that apply to all healthcare practice and might inform a critique. These principles were introduced in Chapter 1 and are: **beneficence** (doing good); **non-maleficence** (avoiding unnecessary harm); **autonomy** (respecting freedom of action) and **justice** (fairness).

Critiquing the ethics of a piece of research is as much about your understanding of what is right, what is wrong and what might be ethically questionable as it is about following a critiquing framework. This is one reason why having an understanding of the Code is important and why you were asked to review it in this chapter.

The discussion and conclusions

The purpose of the discussion and conclusions sections of the paper is to add some context to the results section. Context is achieved by reviewing how well the research has answered the initial question asked (or demonstrated the hypothesis to be true) or not, as well as examining what similar research in the same area has shown and perhaps looking at the policy context within which the findings might operate (Gerrish and Lathlean, 2015).

The discussion also allows the researcher to explain the results that they have found and why they may have arrived at them. The discussion section of a research paper may be presented in one of two ways: it may be a section on its own or it may be contained within the results section with a discussion attached to each of the results. Either style is reasonable.

From the critiquing point of view, there are two common problems that arise in the discussion sections of published research. First, they may be used to expand on the results rather than explain and contextualise them, and second, the discussion of the results may wander away from a discussion of the questions that were originally posed. This final point can be devastating for a paper that has failed to actually address the question it set out to answer. This wandering of the discussion often points to the use of the wrong methodology or data-collection methods, or to the fact that the authors have been distracted from their main aim by incidental, albeit exciting, findings.

Incidental findings that were not part of the original aim of the research can be of questionable value, as the research design, methodology and methods may not support them. That is to say, the incidental findings may be subject to **biases** that the researcher has not anticipated that may mean the findings are of questionable worth.

Theory

By creating a flow diagram of the contents of a research paper it is easy to identify the initial question or hypothesis that the research set out to answer. This can then be used to compare the results identified in the discussion with the initial aims of the study to see if the two are consistent. Not only does this save time but it adds to the clarity of the process (see Figure 3.1).

The discussion section of the paper is also the place where researchers can discuss the limitations of the study that may arise from practical issues with the implementation of research or from issues that were not fully thought out at the start of the study process. Identifying the methodological and other weaknesses of a study in the discussion and conclusions allows the reader to appreciate some of the tensions that present themselves when trying to do research in the real world. The fact that the author identifies issues with the design or implementation of the research should lead them to be a little circumspect over the findings/applicability of their paper; where this is not the case it is certainly worth a mention in the critique!

The best conclusions relate only to the aims of the study and what other research and policy might mean in relation to the findings. It is the nature of nursing and all health and social care research that the findings from a study generate new questions that need answering.

Such questions may arise out of the findings of the research, the lack of definitive findings from the research, or perhaps contradictions between the study and other previous research or existing policy. The diligent researcher will recognise these issues and will suggest areas for further research, which may be presented as questions or general topic areas. Where a paper lacks suggestions for further research it tends to suggest that the researchers have failed to understand the contribution of their paper to the wider understanding of the topic being investigated; the novice nurse might not know what questions should arise following a study, but they can comment when they are not there.

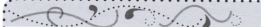

Chapter summary

This chapter has introduced you to the key elements that need to be considered when setting out to undertake a critique of a piece of research and has established why it is important to be able to critique research before considering applying its findings to nursing practice.

There are many methods available to the novice – and, indeed, to the experienced nurse – that help in the process of appraising a piece of research. These include creating an overview and/or flow diagram of the research to highlight important areas and using a critiquing framework to guide the process.

A variety of issues must be considered when critiquing the title of a research paper, including the credentials of the researchers undertaking the study. Sometimes a degree of detective work is necessary in order to critique these in a meaningful way. All researchers should identify the purpose of the research, and its aims or hypotheses, which will inform the choice of research paradigm and methodology chosen for the study.

Ethical considerations are fundamental to all research. Critiquing requires an appreciation of ethical principles as well as consideration of how these are evidenced within the research process. A good discussion section of a paper should identify what the research has shown in relation to its original aims, as well as how these findings reflect what is already known about the subject and the policy context within which the research might be employed in nursing practice.

Activity: Brief outline answer

Activity 3.2: Reflection (page 50)

The first way to quickly ascertain whether a paper is original research is to use the advanced filters that exist in some research engines to ensure that you identify only papers that are empirical research – these are often known as original papers. The second important method is to read the abstract, which will often identify a research aim or question, the methodology used, sampling method applied, data-collection methods used and the key findings, as well as the conclusions of the study. If the elements mentioned here are missing, chances are it is not a research paper.

Further reading

Ellis, P (2016) *Understanding research for nursing students* (3rd edn). London: Sage.

This book provides a structured introduction to research approaches and methods.

Gerrish, K and Lathlean, J (2015) *The research process in nursing* (7th edn). Oxford: Wiley-Blackwell.

Chapter 3 on research ethics is an interesting read.

Moule, P (2015) *Making sense of research in nursing, health and social care* (5th edn). London: Sage.

Chapter 11 on critical appraisal and Appendix 1, a critical appraisal framework, are particularly helpful.

Parahoo, K (2014) *Nursing research: principles, process and issues* (3rd edn). London: Palgrave Macmillan.

Chapter 17 on critiquing research is very helpful.

Useful websites

www.consort-statement.org/consort-statement/overview0 A structured and helpful website that demonstrates clearly strategies for creating research.

www.hra.nhs.uk This is the home of the Human Research Authority for the UK.

Chapter 4
Critiquing research: approach-specific elements

Peter Ellis

NMC Standards for Pre-registration Nursing Education

This chapter will address the following competencies:

Domain 1: Professional values

7. All nurses must be responsible and accountable for keeping their knowledge and skills up to date through continuing professional development. They must aim to improve their performance and enhance the safety and quality of care through evaluation, supervision and appraisal.

9. All nurses must appreciate the value of evidence in practice, be able to understand and appraise research, apply relevant theory and research findings to their work, and identify areas for further investigation.

NMC Essential Skills Clusters

This chapter will address the following ESCs:

Cluster: Care, compassion and communication

1. As partners in the care process, people can trust a newly registered graduate nurse to provide collaborative care based on the highest standards, knowledge and competence.

Cluster: Organisational aspects of care

16. People can trust the newly registered graduate nurse to safely lead, co-ordinate and manage care.

Chapter aims

After reading this chapter, you will be able to:

*   demonstrate an understanding of the important issues for critique within qualitative research;

(Continued)

(Continued)

- demonstrate an understanding of the important issues for critique within quantitative research;
- identify the choices for the different research methods used in qualitative and quantitative research and be able to critique them;
- describe what good data analysis might look like when critiquing qualitative or quantitative research.

Introduction

The purpose of this chapter is to explore in more depth the critical appraisal processes that are applied when critiquing qualitative or quantitative research. The distinction between the two research approaches (or paradigms) has already been made. This chapter will enable you to decipher what good research practice looks like within each of these paradigms and describe some of the reasons for the practical choices made about methodologies and methods within each approach.

The chapter is split into two sections, the first dealing with qualitative research and the second with quantitative research. It complements the critiquing framework in the Appendix to this book and together they identify the questions you might ask of research and some of the answers you might expect from a good paper. As in the previous chapter, there are a number of examples of research included within the text. You may find it useful to have some of these to hand when reading this chapter so that you can engage in critical appraisal of them as you read. Remember as you read this chapter that critiquing is not all about being negative; critique implies identifying the positive aspects of a paper as well as identifying and justifying alternative approaches the researchers might have chosen.

It is important that you understand the research process in order to be able to critique it. To this end we strongly suggest you use at least one, if not more, research textbooks to support your learning and from which to reference your critique. As we shall see later, a good critique will identify something about the research, apply the correct research term to the issue, reference a definition of the term (using a research methods textbook) and then apply the learning about the term to the paper being critiqued.

Critiquing qualitative research

Within this section we will explore the critiquing of qualitative research. Remember, qualitative research asks questions about people's experiences, attitudes, feelings, understandings and opinions. The qualitative paradigm is associated with the social sciences and 'people focused' enquiry; it looks at the world from the point of view of the people who are experiencing or have experienced whatever it is the research is exploring. On the whole, approaches to qualitative research are inductive, that is, they start from a position of neutrality, ask a question and allow the answer to emerge as the research progresses.

Qualitative research is, therefore, concerned with describing and understanding human experiences as they occur and are interpreted in real life. In critiquing qualitative research attention focuses on the **credibility** of the evidence presented as an authentic account and accurate interpretation of the respondents' viewpoints in relation to the research questions being explored. This is in contrast to the attempts within quantitative research to find *the* answer to a given question.

The choice of methodology

We identified in Chapter 3 that the research paradigm upon which a research paper is based has to do with the school of thought upon which it is based. Methodologies are a more detailed plan of action used to undertake the research – the road map, if you like. Within qualitative research the different methodologies provide a structure for undertaking the research and are selected because of how well they actually fit the question asked.

Research summary: choice of methodology

For their study of self-harm in patients with anorexia nervosa, Verschueren et al. (2015) chose to use phenomenology because: *The purpose of a phenomenological research approach is to identify and describe phenomena as perceived by the participants. This method is commonly used to describe a phenomenon which we are aware of but do not fully understand … Phenomenology is concerned with the lived experiences of the participants. It facilitates interaction between the researcher and the participant during data collection and, as a result, makes it possible to gain profound insight into these lived experiences … Therefore, this design is particularly suitable to explore the phenomenon of self-injury in patients with anorexia nervosa* (p64). While this is a perfectly reasonable explanation of, and reason for using, phenomenology for this study, a number of other qualitative methodologies could have been used instead. Given they want to understand the 'lived experience' rather than say generate 'theoretical understanding of', the methodology fits the aim of the study as stated (Ellis, 2016).

Many qualitative research papers do not identify a specific research methodology – they are called **generic** or **exploratory qualitative studies**. This is not, usually, a mistake on the part of the researchers; rather, it is a practical response to the fact that the question they are asking does not fit neatly into one of the established methodologies. In a critique it is often sufficient to point this out and perhaps suggest a methodology that might have been chosen or, alternatively, a means of adjusting the question to make it potentially fit a particular approach with the best critiques suggesting both tweaks to the question and methodologies which fit these.

Table 4.1 shows the main research methodologies used in qualitative research and gives some idea of the type of issues they are used to study.

Research methodologies are, therefore, the overall scheme by which research is undertaken, and the choice of methodology is driven by the exact research question being asked. For example, a question about what it is like to work in an oncology unit, caring for people with cancer, suggests the use of **ethnography**, while developing a theory about how people cope with life with cancer will suggest that the study methodology should be **grounded theory**.

Table 4.1: Potential areas for study and their associated qualitative methodologies	
Methodology	**What it studies**
Ethnography	Studies cultures and groups and how they interact
Grounded theory	Generates, or develops a theory about a social interaction
Phenomenology	Describes the **essence** or perceived reality of an experience
Case study research	Explores case(s) of interest
Generic qualitative	Studies people's attitudes, beliefs, opinions or experiences

When critiquing the choice of methodology chosen for a piece of research it is worth looking at the sometimes subtle differences between the methodologies and perhaps suggesting, rather than categorically stating, how a slightly modified question might have led the researchers to have used a different methodology. Where the methodology chosen appears to fit well with the question being asked, it is important to state why this is the case, as in the example critique earlier. One good method of checking how a topic could be researched is to look at other papers which have examined the same, or similar, topics to see what they have down (and how they have framed their questions); you might find some examples in the literature review/background section of the paper you are critiquing.

Sampling

When critiquing the choice of sampling methods and sample size in qualitative research it is worth remembering what qualitative research seeks to do. Qualitative research seeks to inform the thinking about a topic and seeks for its findings to be potentially **transferable** to other similar situations. This means that the findings are not said to be directly applicable – generalisable – to other similar situations, but they might inform decision-making – especially where the findings are supported by other, similar research.

In **biographic** and **case study** research, the sample may be as few as one individual rising up to dozens in ethnographic research. Most qualitative research methodologies, for example phenomenological or grounded theory research, use sample sizes of between 6 and 15 participants; although this is open to justification by the authors and may also be determined by their findings as they progress through the study.

There are a number of characteristics of qualitative sampling that relate it to the purpose of the topic being studied. Since most qualitative research is about understanding individuals' perceptions and experiences, sampling involves identifying individuals who have had the experience that is being studied. Selecting people because of their common experience is called **purposive sampling** (Streubert and Carpenter, 2010). Because the individuals within the sample are similar on account of the shared experience, the sample may also be said to be **homogeneous**. In qualitative research this is seen as a good feature of the research design, so long as the people selected represent the sorts of people the research question is about.

Homogeneous and purposive sampling means that the findings of qualitative research may be transferable to other similar people in similar situations and contexts – transferability. It is worth noting, however, that just because a sample is said to be homogeneous, this does not mean the interpretation of the experience will be the same for all concerned. Homogeneity in this sense relates to having experienced the same phenomenon; clearly, interpretation of the phenomenon, the individual's own reality, will vary from participant to participant.

Concept summary: purposive sampling

Purposive sampling refers to the fact that individuals are selected because they fit the purpose of the study – their purpose is to be able to talk about whatever phenomenon is being studied. Individuals within such samples are also similar in that they share an experience or some other feature(s) in common; this is referred to as homogeneity, which literally means being the same – at least in respect of one important variable. However, this does not mean that they view the experience in the same way necessarily. When critiquing qualitative samples it is desirable that the characteristics of the individuals in a sample are identified to the reader and that you can understand who has been selected for the study and why. Understanding the characteristics and context of the research aids the reader in understanding how transferable the findings of the study might be to the place that they work and the people that they work with.

Many qualitative studies select participants from groups of individuals who are easily identified and handy to approach. These **convenience samples,** as they are called, are an acceptable way of recruiting participants to study (Parahoo, 2014). When such samples contain individuals who may be vulnerable, it is good practice to show within the sampling how this has been accounted for. Strategies may include approaching the individuals through a third party (such as another member of staff that they know, or a relative or friend), seeking consent via a partner or close relative or just excluding people who lack the ability to consent freely from the study.

Vulnerability may also lie in dependent relationships between the researcher and the subject, for example a nurse and patient, or a lecturer and student. Care will need to be exercised in the consent process in such circumstances to avoid claims of coercion. Again using a third party to recruit and consent people in these circumstances is good practice and would be worthy of a positive comment in any critique.

Example critique: purposive and convenience sampling

In their study of the lived experiences of diabetes among elderly, rural-dwelling people, George and Thomas (2010, p1094) used *a purposive sample … drawn from local agencies on ageing … English speaking people aged 65–85 years … all confined to their homes and living in a rural area … with diabetes*. It is clear from their description that all of the participants were selected to suit the purposes of the research *to elucidate experiences and perceptions of self-management of their diabetes as narrated by older people with insulin-dependent diabetes living in a rural area* (George and Thomas, 2010, p1094). Evidently, the sample included only English-speaking people and those willing to discuss their disease; this will limit the transferability of the findings, but it is a reasonable practical way of sampling in qualitative research. The identification of people via local agencies that care for the elderly demonstrates that this is a convenience sample. Being a convenience sample raises some questions about whether the participants felt coerced into participating in order to please the care agencies.

Activity 4.1   *Reflection*

Reflect on how you respond to approaches for help or information from different people. What factors influence the responses that you give and in what situations do you feel more obliged to comply with the request? How might this reflect in the ways in which people respond to requests to become involved in research in the hospital or other clinical setting?

An outline answer is provided at the end of the chapter.

Many qualitative studies use the point of **data saturation** as an idealised way of determining the size of the sample to be studied. Data from the interview or focus groups are analysed as the study progresses, and recruitment stops when no new ideas are emerging from the data – that is, when the data is **saturated** (Macnee and McCabe, 2008). This is a very reasonable approach to use in qualitative research and may be positively critiqued.

One other common approach to sampling, which is frequently used in grounded theory, is called **theoretical sampling** (Glaser and Strauss, 1967). Theoretical sampling occurs when the researcher has analysed early interviews within the study and has started to create some initial theories. This analysis leads the researcher to ask additional questions and prompts them to purposively recruit further participants to the study who are suitable to help answer emerging questions or to firm up the emerging theory. This is an extension of the idea of data saturation and makes good sense within qualitative methodologies which are inductive – that is which allow the findings to emerge from the study as the data are collected, rather than starting with a preconceived idea as to what the findings might be.

The best qualitative research papers will therefore identify the characteristics of their sample, the recruitment and sampling method used as well as demonstrating how they have tried to go about this process in an ethical manner.

The choice of data-collection methods

Methods refer to the tools used to collect the data for a research project. When critiquing data-collection methods within qualitative research, it is important, as ever, to bear in mind the purpose of the research (which arises from the research question), the chosen methodology, and the capabilities and vulnerabilities of the people being researched. The nature of the research question will strongly determine the sense of the data-collection method being used.

Within qualitative research there are four main approaches to data collection: interviews, focus groups, observation and examination of artefacts. The choice of the data-collection method will relate strongly not only to the topic under investigation but also to the characteristics of the participants.

For example, it might be reasonable to question a qualitative study that enquired into the nature of a potentially embarrassing topic (such as sexually transmitted diseases) using a focus group. It is clearly more appropriate (regardless of the methodology) to ask such questions in a one-to-one interview.

Example critique: data collection using focus groups

In designing the focus group approach for their study of emotional well-being support in high schools, Kendal et al. (2011) provided a few strategies to help overcome some of the issues which may have caused participants not to engage. For example they used **vignettes** so that the participants could talk about their own experience of needing emotional support as if they were talking about the person in the vignette. They tried to overcome the fear of identification in the research by not collecting participants' names. So while focus groups are not always the best way to collect data about sensitive topics, such as mental health, nor are they always the best method for use with teenagers, Kendal et al. demonstrate they have thought about this and tried to minimise the impact of the threats to focus group data collection within their study.

Where there are potential power relationships, or when individuals may be vulnerable in other ways, it may not be appropriate to use focus groups or observations to collect qualitative data – even if methodologically this is the preferred data-collection method. In these instances the usefulness of the chosen methods has to take second place to the ethical principles of avoiding harm and respecting autonomy.

Activity 4.2   *Critical thinking*

In what sorts of situations might you feel less able to speak your mind than others? Why is this and why might this answer help you to understand how research participants view data-collection methods in qualitative research?

There are some possible answers at the end of the chapter.

Observational data collection may be a benefit in studies seeking to find out what people do or how they behave in certain situations. The use of observation may not be the correct method when the purpose of the study is to understand an issue from the perspective of the participant. Observation just does not fit the purpose – it is used to see what people do rather than study what they think. Observation followed by interviews or a focus group discussion, however, may be an appropriate choice of method when the research is seeking to understand what people do and why they do it in a particular situation.

In some research methodologies, for example ethnography, there is a clear need for the use of multiple methods of data collection. Ethnography seeks to understand the culture (beliefs, shared understandings and values) as well as the behaviours within a group; this requires a mix of observation, participation in the group and interviews (Parahoo, 2014). Some ethnography may also include the examination of artefacts such as pictures and letters in an effort to understand their meaning to the group. Failure to undertake at least two levels of data collection within ethnography would give cause for concern and raise questions about the completeness of the data collection.

Some questions around data collection in the qualitative methodologies are somewhat more subtle. For example, there remain questions about the use of semi-structured interviews in phenomenology where the consensus view used to be that the interviews should be unstructured (so that the respondent can shape the direction of the conversation). In many critical appraisals it would be reasonable to point this out without committing to one argument or the other.

Critiquing qualitative research methods, therefore, requires the reviewer to make some judgement about the justification that the researcher has made for their choice of methods. It also requires the reviewer to ask questions of themselves about what approach they would use when trying to obtain the same sorts of information from people in similar circumstances.

The analysis and results

The data that are produced in qualitative research are words. These words need sorting, grouping and interpreting in order to help make sense of the data collected for a study. There are several stages that can add credibility and **rigour** to this process and demonstrate the researcher's commitment to producing research findings that are transparent and high quality.

Concept summary: credibility and rigour

Credibility refers to how believable a piece of qualitative research is. The use of the term in relation to qualitative research suggests the research undertaken actually answers what it set out to answer because of the quality of the way in which the research has been done.

Rigour in qualitative research suggests the research process has been undertaken in a well-thought through, fully explained and transparent manner. It also requires this is fully explained to those reading the paper.

There is no single right way in which to examine qualitative data. What is always important in qualitative data analysis is that the process is well explained and the decisions made in the process appear logical and transparent (credible and rigorous). This transparency requires the paper to explain exactly how the data were analysed and by whom, and what strategies they put in place to confirm the conclusions they came to.

It should be apparent the study has been conducted in a neutral manner and the findings have been allowed to emerge – that is, the whole research process has been inductive and not based on confirming a pre-existing hypothesis. This neutrality of the data analysis process is said to bring **confirmability** to the study (Polit and Beck, 2008).

Commonly, papers will say that the author(s) read and reread the data (usually **verbatim** transcripts of interviews or focus groups) looking for common ideas and themes identifying the issues that were most important to the participants. This is a reasonable approach to data analysis, although many qualitative researchers are now using computer programs. What is important in critiquing the analysis of qualitative research is not so much the strategy used but the supplementary strategies used to check the credibility and trustworthiness of this initial data analysis approach.

Key among the strategies used to confirm the findings of a study are the use of a second person to review the data collected – be they transcripts of interviews or focus groups, video or notes from observations of other artefacts – and come to their own conclusions about the findings. There may be some discussion about how a consensus view about the study results was then arrived at. A good study should explain this process in enough detail for the reader to understand what was done, by whom, and when, so the reader is content about both the the rigour and credibility of the analysis process.

The best studies using a single method (such as interviews or focus groups) will further check, and report on, the credibility of their findings in one of two ways. The first is to return the results to some, if not all, of the participants asking the question 'Is this interpretation of the interview a good representation of what you said?' The second approach is to present the findings to other researchers, or people with a special knowledge of the area of investigation, who are encouraged to ask probing questions about the methods used and the findings arrived at (Polit and Beck, 2013). Failure to do either of these might lead to some critical discussion in the critique.

In studies employing more than one data-collection method the consistency of the findings between the different data-collection methods may be used to demonstrate the degree of credibility of the research. Where more than one data collector is used or different approaches employed, the study should demonstrate a consistency in the data collection; this is termed **dependability**.

A further strategy that helps the reader understand and perhaps come to some agreement with the findings of qualitative research is the use of verbatim (that is, word-for-word) quotes from the participants of the research alongside the themes and categories identified by the researcher. This allows the reader to understand how they have arrived at the findings they have and to develop an awareness of why the researchers have come to the conclusions they have. Clearly, the interpretation of what a research participant has said relies to some extent on the context of the conversation in which they said it; nevertheless, verbatim quotes give the critical reviewer a view into the world of the research participant that is missing in studies that do not use them.

Example critique: establishing credibility

In their study of emergency room nurses' perceptions and experiences of caring for older people, Gallagher et al. (2014) used focus groups for data collection. Two researchers independently coded the data using a framework and verbatim quotes are presented in the article. While both of these strategies are useful in helping demonstrate rigour and credibility, there is no real information about the process undertaken when the researchers met to discuss the emerging themes nor does it appear that participants were asked to verify the findings of the focus group either at the end of the session or subsequently. While neither of these issues mean the study is poor, they are both worth a mention in any critique.

While the findings of qualitative research are not said to be generalisable (necessarily applicable) to other people similar to the participants, the existence in the discussion of other similar research showing similar findings demonstrates the study has some transferability to other groups of individuals.

Critiquing quantitative research

Quantitative research is research that uses numbers and statistics; it is concerned with cause and effect, exposures and outcomes. Key among the concerns for quantitative research are that it should be **valid**, **reliable** and **generalisable**.

Concept summary: validity, reliability and generalisability

Validity is the ability of a data-collecting tool (a method) to measure what it is supposed to be measuring. For example, we know that a sphygmomanometer (when used properly) will measure blood pressure; however, it is much more difficult to know how well a questionnaire designed to measure anxiety levels actually does so because it may be hard to define what anxiety is. In many studies of anxiety and stress the data collected from questionnaires are supplemented by taking biological samples and measuring the level of cortisol (a hormone associated with stress) in them, as a way of validating the findings.

Reliability refers to the reproducibility of the results of the study. Reliability may refer to whether the data-collection tool (such as a questionnaire) produces broadly similar results when used again in the same population, when applied to the same sample at a different time or when the tool is used by another researcher.

Generalisability refers to the extent to which the findings from a piece of research can be extended out to the general population of people in a similar position – that is, whether the sample used in the research is representative enough of the population to which the findings of the research are to be applied.

Many quantitative studies focus on answering a question that is posed as a hypothesis, which we described earlier as being an idea that can be tested using the scientific method. By their nature quantitative studies are therefore **deductive**, setting out to answer the question of the research using a methodology and methods best suited to establishing the truth, or otherwise, of the initial hypothesis.

The choice of methodology

As with all research, the methodology (which is the broad plan of action for the study) has to fit the questions being asked. The wrong choice of methodology means a study cannot answer the questions it set out to answer. When critiquing the choice of methodology it is important to understand what each of the different methodologies can be used to research. For example, cause and effect can only be examined with any confidence in experimental studies (which include randomised controlled trials) and cohort studies as these are **prospective** and **longitudinal** (that is, they collect data as things happen over a period of time). Quantitative methods that are not both prospective and longitudinal cannot make this claim as they do not collect data in a forward-going real-time manner.

Table 4.2 shows the sorts of questions that the various quantitative methodologies can be used to answer.

While Table 4.2 is not an exhaustive list of the quantitative methodologies, it provides some clarity as to what the different methods can do. In terms of critiquing the choice of quantitative research methodologies, perhaps the most important question is whether the chosen approach is suitable for examining cause-and-effect relationships.

Table 4.2: Questions that different quantitative methodologies can be used to answer	
Questions	**Methodology**
If x is done, what will happen? If x is done, how often will y happen?	Experiment/quasi-experiment/ randomised controlled trial.
If a person is exposed to x, will they develop outcome (disease) y? Does exposure to x cause outcome y?	Cohort studies.
What exposure x might have caused this individual to have outcome y?	Case-control studies.
In this group of people how many have been exposed to x or have outcome y? What is the prevalence of x or y in this group?	Cross-sectional studies.
The data show that when x increases in the population so too does y. Might they be associated? When exposure x increases and outcome y increases is there potential that the two are associated in some way?	Ecological studies.
Source: Ellis, 2016.	

This is perhaps best understood by remembering that all quantitative methodologies are concerned with the quality of the measurement of variables, where variables are any factors within a study that may differ (vary) between study participants. The quality of the measurements, and therefore the validity and reliability of the study, relies heavily on the elimination of bias within the research process.

Concept summary: bias

Bias is defined as a deviation from the truth. Bias occurs when a deviation from the truth is the result of defects in the way in which a study is carried out. For example, **recall bias** occurs where a study relies on the memory of participants, for example remembering what they ate last week, recalling their alcohol intake over a period of time or whether or not they have ever had chickenpox.

Because, in the examples given, these variables are not being measured in real time (prospectively) or over a period of time (longitudinally) or, indeed, in a standardised way (which will affect both validity and reliability), there is a degree of uncertainty about how good the quality of the data collected actually is. Significantly bias can mean a study is fatally flawed and its findings are of no value; consequently quantitative researchers expend a lot of time and energy trying to design bias out of their studies.

Taking these issues into account identifies why studies that seek to prove cause and effect need to be prospective and longitudinal, while those that seek only to measure the amount of a certain variable or demonstrate an association or correlation (which conceptually are not as strong as demonstrating cause-and-effect relationships) do not.

Example critique: choice of methodology

Williams et al. (2009) set out to investigate – using a validated personality assessment questionnaire – personality differences specifically related to caring between a group of female staff nurses and a group of female controls. They chose a case-control study as they wanted to look at the differences in personality but were not trying to show a cause-and- effect relationship – merely an association.

This is a reasonable choice of methodology: it would not be possible to show that a more caring disposition creates the desire to be a nurse as the study did not take place before the staff nurses joined the nursing profession and it may be that being a nurse has made the nurse more caring than their non-nursing peers.

When critiquing the choice of methodology, therefore, it is important to identify the expressed purpose (aims and objectives) of the study and the level of proof associated with it. Identifying the purpose of the study will indicate whether the methodology needs to be prospective and longitudinal or not. A good critique will pick up on this and might express that the choice of study methodology is a good one, a poor one or that alternative methodologies might have been chosen.

Sampling

When thinking about the quality of the sampling methods applied in quantitative research, it is important to remember that the key purpose of this form of enquiry is to produce data that are generalisable. That is to say, quantitative studies seek to produce results that can be applied beyond the sample in which the study took place. To be generalisable, therefore, quantitative studies need to have samples that are **representative** of people who are broadly similar to all the people the study is about.

> **Concept summary: representativeness**
>
> Representativeness is about the degree to which the study sample is comparable to the population from which it was taken (for example, in relation to gender, age, ethnicity and severity of disease). The more typical the sample is with regard to the population the study is about, the more likely the findings of the study hold true in that population (generalisability).

In terms of critiquing, this means that the sample used for the study should represent the sorts of people who are identified in the study question. For example, a study of the understanding of dietary management among people newly diagnosed with diabetes should identify what it means by diabetes (type 1 or type 2) as well as what it means by newly diagnosed (say, in the last six months). The selection of potential participants for the study would then be focused on all people who fit these criteria; this would be termed the **study population**.

In some research, all the people in this population might be studied, especially when the population is drawn from a small geographic area or from people with a rare disease – that is, assuming they all consented to participate. Studies that employ this type of sample might include **cross-sectional studies**.

In more sophisticated studies, such as experimental studies, the selection of people from a large potential study population allows everyone the same chance of being included in the study. This is called **probability sampling** and produces a **study sample**. If the sample size is large enough (as calculated using statistical formulae), it can produce a sample that is representative of the larger population – and hence generalisable results.

Where a paper does not identify the processes that occurred in relation to forming the study sample, there are questions that need to be asked about the quality of the sampling, the potential for the introduction of bias and therefore about how generalisable the findings of such research can be.

Activity 4.3   *Critical thinking*

If someone were to undertake a study looking at stress in nurses, consider how many of your colleagues they might need to sample in order to get a reasonable understanding of this issue. Consider what impression they might form of stress in nursing if they were to interview just one or two of your colleagues perhaps directly after a night shift.

An outline answer is provided at the end of the chapter.

In **randomised controlled trials** (RCTs) the process goes a step further. Because RCTs seek to examine the difference in outcomes between two or more similar groups to investigate the effectiveness of an intervention, there is a need for the two groups to be broadly similar at the start of the study – or any findings made could be claimed to be the result of the differences between the groups rather than the results of the intervention being studied. So in an RCT you would expect to see the study sample is further divided into cases (participants to whom the intervention/study drug is given) and controls (participants who get a dummy intervention or drug) (Ellis, 2016). This process must happen randomly (to avoid introducing **selection bias** to the study) and all good RCTs will identify how this is achieved.

Example critique: randomised sample

In their study of supporting weight loss through providing all meals versus providing advice, Mellor et al. (2013) randomised participants using an online randomisation generator. The method used ensured equal numbers in each arm of the study and ensured an even split of genders between the two groups. Mellor et al. (2014, p378) explained that 'Participants were volunteers recruited by advertisement from both the University of Hull and the local area'. In terms of critique, one might comment that people who have a connection with the university may be different in some ways to members of the local population and that perhaps this ought to have been accounted for in the design of the randomisation.

In some cases where the splitting of the groups cannot happen randomly, there remain questions about the quality of the research process, especially around the introduction of bias. While it would be correct to critique this element of the research, allowances have to be made where the decision not to create the groups randomly was a practical consideration – for example, when it is hard to hide from the participants and the researchers which group the individual participant has been allocated to; for example when using a particular type of wound dressing.

In case-control studies the selection of cases is based on them having the outcome (usually a disease) of interest with controls being similar in as many other respects as possible (for example, age, gender, ethnicity, income group and educational attainment). In matched cohort studies the controls are chosen because they are similar to the cases being studied in as many respects as possible other than being exposed to the potential cause of the disease under study. In both types of study it is the role of the researcher to create a convincing argument as to why they chose the control groups they did, and the best papers will identify the limitations of the study that arise from the compromises made in this process somewhere in the discussion. Regardless of whether the authors identify the limitation or not, the best critiques will identify and discuss these issues.

Many quantitative papers identify a starting sample but appear to report data from a smaller sample in the results. This is usually the result of losses to the study from people withdrawing for any number of reasons. It is reasonable to criticise a study in which this occurs when the reasons for, and the characteristics of, the withdrawals are not discussed. There are good reasons for this.

Some withdrawals may be related to some aspect of the thing being studied, for example, a side effect of a drug. Significant numbers of withdrawals from a study because of a side effect may not have statistical, but may have important clinical, implications. Withdrawal of certain groups of people from the study, perhaps older patients or those of a particular gender, may mean that the findings of the study are skewed and that they can no longer claim to be generalisable. Clearly, in a study of two arms such as an RCT, significant withdrawals from the treatment arm may mean that the new drug or intervention is unacceptable to many people and may not be as clinically successful as the researchers suggest. This is worthy of an unambiguous negative critique.

The choice of data-collection methods

We have already made the assertion that all quantitative methodologies are concerned with the quality of the measurement of variables. Nowhere within the quantitative research process is this more obvious than in the choice of data-collection methods. Essentially, there are two elements to data-collection methods that are open to potential critique. The first is the actual choice of the tool itself and its potential to be able to measure whatever it is that it is trying to measure – its validity. Second is the issue of how the tool is actually put to work, how reliable the way in which it was used is.

The most frequently used data-collection tools used in nursing research are questionnaires and other forms of surveys. In many cases the variables that a study seeks to measure are already the subjects of well-tried and tested questionnaires, or other tools, the validity of which is well established. The best research papers will identify why they chose the questionnaire(s) and how well these might apply to the people they are studying. Poorer quality papers will identify what tools they used but give little or no explanation as to why. A top tip for critiquing is to look up the tool online and see what other researchers might say about its strengths and weaknesses; the very best critiques might go so far as to identify alternative data-collection tools.

Activity 4.4   *Research and finding out*

There are a large number of questionnaires that exist to measure diverse health and socially related variables in research. These tools can be used to measure variables such as quality of life, mental well-being and levels of anxiety either generally or in relation to specific diseases. Go online and try to identify some of these and read about what it is they

continued ...

are designed to be able to measure. Spend some time trying to find some critiques of the strengths and weaknesses of the particular tool and alternative tools one might use to investigate a variable you are interested in, for example quantifying pain. You may find this approach useful when critiquing a paper.

There are some websites identified at the end of this chapter where you could go to look at some validated questionnaires and data-collection tools.

Other data for quantitative studies may be collected from existing sources such as databases and medical and nursing records. The quality of this data will vary greatly and the best studies will make allowances for this and may make some efforts to check the quality of both the data and the accuracy and consistency (reliability) of the collection of it for research purposes (especially where more than one person is used for data collection).

Physiological and biological data are frequently collected in quantitative studies. The quality of these forms of data is thought by many nurses to be beyond question; this is not, however, always the case. For example, blood pressure measurements, even when undertaken using the same apparatus, vary between individuals. The best quality research will try to minimise this difference by training all those involved to use the same method to take blood pressures and thereby increase reliability.

With regard to biological and physiological data, the best papers will record how specimens and measurements were taken, by whom, under what conditions, where, how often and how data-collection staff were trained. In some of the best research reports there will be data on the degree of agreement between different data-collection staff, typically measured in statistical terms. When critiquing, if this level of detail is missing it is worthy of comment.

The analysis and results

The analysis of quantitative research invariably requires the use of statistics. These statistics are of two separate kinds. The first are **descriptive statistics**, the purpose of which is to describe the study sample and perhaps some of the outcomes. The best research papers will contain descriptive statistics that explain the frequency, spread and measures of central tendency (for example, the **means** and **medians**) of the data. Such data should give you a good idea of some of the characteristics of the study participants, such as their ages and gender. In comparison studies such as RCTs and matched cohorts, the reader should also be able to see that the two groups are broadly similar in all described variables at the start of the study – if they appear not to be so, this would give cause for critique.

The second form of statistics used are what are referred to as **inferential statistics**. These statistics describe the levels of confidence that the researchers place in their findings and are derived from applying various statistical tests.

There are a large number of statistical tests that can be applied to numerical data, and the best papers leave the reader in no doubt about what tests have been applied using which statistical packages. Clearly, it is beyond the scope of this text to delve into these now; however, there are many good guides that explain which statistical tests apply to which forms of data and in what circumstances.

Activity 4.5   *Research and finding out*

There are a large number of statistical tests that can be applied to numerical data. Go online and try to identify some of these and read about what it is they are designed to do. You may find this strategy useful when critiquing a paper.

There are some websites identified at the end of this chapter where you could look at examples of statistics used with different forms of data.

The analysis and presentation of results within quantitative research can be quite confusing because of the numbers involved. The best papers will, however, present their findings in a variety of ways including graphs, tables and charts, many of which are fairly simple to understand and interpret. It is not a matter for critique that the reader is not familiar with the approach to analysis employed. A good critique will involve the novice reader in learning some things about the basic elements of what they are reading and applying it.

Chapter summary

The approach to critiquing either research paradigm is driven by what the research ultimately aims to do. The choice of research methodology, and whether or not it is qualitative or quantitative, should have been informed by the exact questions, the nature of those questions and the type of person about whom the research seeks to find answers.

There are various approaches to identifying and recruiting samples for both qualitative and quantitative research, and these are driven by both theoretical and practical issues. Similarly, there are a number of different methods that can be used to collect data, and it is the role of the researcher to defend the choices they made.

As with all stages of the research process, the choice of data-collection method arises out of both theoretical and practical considerations. Researchers need to make it plain why they make the choices they do. While recognising this, a good critique may include some suggestions about why the method might or might not be the best choice, as well as suggestions for other methods of data collection.

The analysis of data is a process that needs justification in the qualitative paradigm, and explanation and transparency in both qualitative and quantitative research.

Activities: Brief outline answers

Activity 4.1: Reflection (page 64)

The ways in which we are approached and by whom certainly have an effect on the ways in which we respond to requests for help. We feel obligations to people that employ us, people who we work with and our family. These obligations arise from a sense of duty, belonging and, in the case of family, love, and may conflict with our own true wishes. Approaches in person are harder to ignore, while those in writing or via e-mail may prove easier to ignore. Whilst writing this answer I was phoned by someone collecting for a charity I do not want to support; it was easy to say no on the phone, whereas face-to-face in the street I might spend more time over saying no.

Asking people who are patients to become involved in research may create dilemmas for them where they, too, feel a sense of obligation arising out of duty to respond to the care they have received, the desire to belong and please their carers, and perhaps affection and gratitude. As suggested in the text, this may mean that researchers have to explore ways for patient participants to exercise freedom of choice in relation to research, which may mean making it easy to say no or simply ignore a written request.

Activity 4.2: Critical thinking (page 65)

There are often potential issues within qualitative research that need to be accounted for in the choice of data-collection methods. These include power relationships between the researcher and the participant – and, indeed, between participants themselves. For instance, you may not feel able to talk openly about how you feel about your job in front of your boss and you may not want to talk about your home life in front of your colleagues.

Similarly, participants in research are not likely to want to discuss certain issues in a focus group format, and if they do, they may choose not to be completely truthful, so the choice of method will impact on the credibility of the research findings.

Activity 4.3: Critical thinking (page 72)

If researchers were to only interview a couple of nurses as they came off a night shift it is likely they would form the impression that nurses were all terribly stressed, or perhaps not. The impression they would form would be influenced almost entirely by what sort of night the two nurses had experienced; in this respect it is influenced by the timing of the study and the fact only two nurses are involved.

Further reading

Bland, M (2015) *An introduction to medical statistics* (4th edn). Oxford: Oxford University Press.

A really well-known and comprehensive beginners' guide to statistics.

Coughlan, M, Cronin, P and Ryan, F (2007) Step-by-step guide to critiquing research. Part 1: quantitative research. *British Journal of Nursing,* 16 (11): 658–63.

This is a reasonable overview of critiquing quantitative research.

Ellis, P (2016) *Understanding research for nursing students* (3rd edn). London: Sage.

A student's guide to research.

Parahoo, K (2014) *Nursing research: principles, process and issues* (3rd edn). London: Palgrave Macmillan.

Chapter 17 on critiquing research is very helpful.

Ryan, F, Coughlan, M and Cronin, P (2007) Step-by-step guide to critiquing research. Part 2: qualitative research. *British Journal of Nursing,* 16 (12): 738–44.

This is a reasonable overview of critiquing qualitative research.

Silverman, D (2009) *Doing qualitative research: a practical handbook* (3rd edn). London: Sage.

A good guide to undertaking qualitative research.

Useful websites

http://statpages.org A very useful statistics resource.

www.graphpad.com Click on 'Visit the Data Analysis Resource Center' and explore the various headings in the statistics guide.

www.dummies.com/how-to/education-languages/math/statistics.html A fun and easy to use website full of information about statistics.

Websites containing validated data-collection questionnaires

www.healthmeasurement.org/Measures.html A website with links to and descriptions of a number of widely used validated questionnaires.

www.sf-36.org/ Short form 36 is widely used to measure self-reported quality of life and functionality.

Chapter 5
Making sense of subjective experience

Lioba Howatson-Jones and Peter Ellis

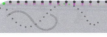

NMC Standards for Pre-registration Nursing Education

This chapter will address the following competencies:

Domain 1: Professional values

9. All nurses must appreciate the value of evidence in practice, be able to understand and appraise research, apply relevant theory and research findings to their work, and identify areas for further investigation.

Domain 3: Nursing practice and decision-making

1. All nurses must use up-to-date knowledge and evidence to assess, plan, deliver and evaluate care, communicate findings, influence change and promote health and best practice. They must make person-centred, evidence-based judgements and decisions, in partnership with others involved in the care process, to ensure high-quality care.

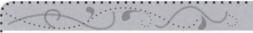

NMC Essential Skills Clusters

This chapter will address the following ESCs:

Cluster: Care, compassion and communication

3. People can trust the newly registered graduate nurse to respect them as individuals and strive to help them to preserve their dignity at all times.

Chapter aims

After reading this chapter, you will be able to:

*   identify how subjective experience relates to other forms of evidence;
*   understand the role of subjective experience in the interpretation of evidence;
*   discuss particular stances that might be adopted;
*   contextualise lived experience.

Introduction

This chapter explains how subjective experience needs to be considered alongside objective and more rational and empirical forms of evidence. It will help you to start making sense of your experiences identifying how these might fit with other forms of evidence. The chapter addresses questions of why it might be that in an era of scientific certainty and effectiveness, professionals feel increasingly anxious and uncertain about the delivery of care and patients feel increasingly uncared for. It is important that healthcare does not become objectified as 'something' we do to others as opposed to recognising it as something we do *with* 'someone' and that a range of evidence is utilised to support practice, taking account of objective knowledge and more subjective experience as appropriate.

The chapter begins by exploring subjective experience from the perspective of the nurse as well as of the patient. This experience is then related to other forms of evidence such as objective data, research findings and audit. The role subjectivity still plays in the interpretation and implementation of rational knowledge is considered further and related to the stances that may be adopted. The chapter closes by contextualising the lived experience of practitioners in relation to making sense of the multiple dimensions of the evidence base which they may use to inform practice.

Subjective experience

Subjective experience can be defined as how we make sense of a situation, how it affects us individually and what we feel about it. We learn from the experiences we have because through interaction with our physical and social environment, we develop knowledge (this notion of experiential evidence is reflected in Figure 1.1 in Chapter 1 (p21) as one of the influences on practice). This knowledge may be modified as we encounter and respond to different situations. Such knowledge may be consciously considered when thinking **cognitively** and reflectively about what is taking place. However, sometimes we are not aware of the learning taken from experiences until it emerges as intuitive knowing – what some people call secondary knowledge.

Intuitive knowledge is difficult to articulate precisely because there is a lack of awareness of its existence – only that the nurse seems to 'sense' what to do in practice. Subjective experience and subjective knowledge are influenced, in part, by our histories, our ability to reflect as well as cultural understanding.

Benner's (1984) study of the development and progression of nursing knowledge identified intuitive knowing as an essential part of the advancing practice of the experienced nurse. This means in complex situations the experienced nurse is able to identify solutions to problems that are difficult to explain but they know to be right, for example, dealing with emergencies or recognising unusual features within routine practice. Intuition and empathy form a part of such experiential knowing that is not easily rationalised, more tentative and, therefore, uncertain (Heron, 1996). Such abstractions have been called 'sixth sense, instinct and gut feeling' (Muir, 2004, p50). Benner's (1984) work and that of Muir (2004) are founded on the principle that intuition resulting from experience provides a substantial evidence base for practice. This contrasts with more analytical approaches that consider the evidence surrounding experience and actions taken in order to substantiate the knowledge used. Consider the following case study to identify how this might work in practice.

Case study: Detecting a case of tracheal stricture

*Anja had been involved in a motorcycle accident while on holiday in Cyprus, where she had sustained extensive head injuries. These had left her in a **vegetative state**, although she was able to breathe on her own through a **tracheostomy tube** with supplementary oxygen. Anja had been transferred back to a hospital in the UK for assessment and the planning of her ongoing care. She was not suitable for admission to an intensive care unit or a high-dependency ward as her condition was categorised as chronic rather than acute, but Anja still required special nursing, particularly at night. Consequently, a number of flexi nurses were drafted in to help with her care.*

*During a night shift Maureen – the nurse on duty – noticed that Anja seemed restless and 'just did not look right'. Anja's **vital signs** and **pulse oximetry** that Maureen recorded were within normal parameters for Anja, and there was no apparent incontinence or reason for discomfort as she was nursed on an airflow pressure mattress. Maureen decided to check the tracheostomy tube, first undertaking tracheal suction and then changing the tube, even though the pulse oximeter reading was normal. Anja remained restless.*

Maureen was still not happy with Anja's condition although she could not account for this. Maureen asked the anaesthetist to come and review Anja. The anaesthetist, who was relatively inexperienced, examined Anja and also could not find anything specific but called other medical colleagues for their opinion. By this stage an hour had elapsed and Maureen noticed a sudden significant drop in Anja's pulse oximetry reading to well below the normal reading, which would, within the pulse oximetry guidelines, have signalled the need to call for medical assistance. By this time the medical consensus had already been reached to take Anja to theatre.

*When Anja arrived in the anaesthetic room her respiration rate had climbed dramatically and she had emptied her bowels – another potential sign of stress. Anja was in theatre for some time where it was discovered that she had a 60 per cent stricture of her trachea (**tracheal stricture**). Because of the supplementary oxygen, this had not been reflected in the pulse oximetry recording, which measured the level of oxygen saturation of haemoglobin and not the effectiveness of pulmonary ventilation. Had Maureen relied only on the pulse oximeter readings to assess Anja's well-being, it might have taken longer for Anja to receive the medical intervention she needed. Maureen's experience had taught her to look at her patient as well as the physiological data, and to take note of her intuitive promptings.*

The case study illustrates the benefits of nurses integrating their subjective impressions with the available objective data to enhance patient care. Combining subjective knowledge of the person with the analysis of physiological data obtained (e.g. Anja's pulse oximetry readings and respiration rate) is an important part of nursing practice. The subjective element of this integration of knowledge is gained from seeing and examining the person/patient as well as communicating with them and taking note of interactive information. Sometimes the strength of practitioner opinion is enhanced by a consensus decision when other professionals are consulted, in order to ascertain whether they have come to the same conclusions given the same information (for more on this, see Chapter 6).

Making sense of subjective evidence is a part of developing as a nurse and in your understanding of what it means to *nurse*. Learning a skill means transforming information into embedded knowledge, which is manifested through intuitive and skilled action – what some call *craftsmanship* (Sennett, 2008). Learning the *craft* of nursing will inevitably be based on your personal experiences, opportunities and motivations, such as curiosity to find out more, which develops into the practical knowledge of nursing – what some call the *professional craft* (Titchen et al., 2004, p108). You will have noticed in life how some people are more curious than others and develop an understanding of various things, both professional and more day-to-day, not because they are particularly clever, but because they are inquisitive. In the sense discussed here, nurses need to both experience situations and be inquisitive enough to learn from them in order to develop their professional craftsmanship; it is not enough just to experience, you also need to question. Consider the following case study to understand the role of subjectivity in the development of practice.

Case study: Sunitta's developing practice

Sunitta was in the first year of her nurse preparation programme and was trying to develop her practice. She had little experience in care settings, but came from a large extended family with whom she interacted a lot. Sunitta's mentor was impressed with her ability to develop a therapeutic relationship with her patients. Sunitta would introduce herself and, with an easy manner, find out what they needed most. As she became more confident, Sunitta was able to deal with more challenging situations such as working with a confused patient. However, Sunitta found it difficult to deconstruct what she did so fluently in practice in order to identify what it was that she did and ways of further improving it.

In order to provide evidence of how she was developing her practice of establishing therapeutic relationships, Sunitta needed to find a way to demonstrate how her practice was changing. Sunitta made use of a reflective approach that allowed her to use stories of her practice, which she then examined through reflective writing (see Reflective Practice in Nursing *also in this series to find out more about this). Critically examining these stories in relation to communication theory helped Sunitta to develop her understanding of possible alternative strategies that she might use should the situation demand it. She also became clearer about how her communication responses were triggered and what she found difficult, which was a first step to being able to employ alternative strategies.*

Discussing her practice experiences with others during an **action learning set** *on her return to university helped Sunitta to identify some further ways of responding that some of her peers had used. One peer had needed to deal with conflict when a patient became very angry. Sunitta found this account especially helpful as she knew that conflict was something she avoided. She decided to return to the literature to find out more and to talk to her mentor about this the next time she was in practice.*

This case study helps to illustrate the importance of recognising the contribution of personal as well as professional experiences in the development of subjective knowledge for practice. Private and professional knowledge interrelate and continue to develop and become transformed as they become integrated, informing each other and making something new. Nevertheless, it is also important to validate this knowledge. Sunitta did this by reading communication literature and through discussion with her mentor. This is important in order to be able to articulate new knowledge.

You might find it easier to consider the development of self and the knowledge which you have as being like a giant jigsaw. You take all the experiences and understandings you have and try to create a giant picture of what you know; you do this by testing new experiences against what you know, or what you think you know. Sometimes you discard old knowledge or understandings and sometimes you reject new knowledge and understandings; however you can only safely do this by reflecting on experiences and testing them against other forms of understanding either alone (e.g. by reflection and seeking further information) or with others (e.g. in group discussion, teaching or action learning sets). However you proceed, you start to build up a picture of the world from your own point of view with your own understandings, and as you become more questioning, you understand there are bits of the picture missing; you use the influences on practice modified by the dispositions of the evidence-based nurse (see Figure 1.1 on p21), which includes reflection, to continue to fill in these gaps, while understanding that the picture will never be finished.

What patients find helpful in the relationships they build with nurses is not always easy to research and therefore the evidence of what works must be subjectively grasped (Baines, 1998). Developing relationships for good practice can relate to how cared for individuals feel themselves to be. It is of note that despite increasing scientific certainty, some recent patient experiences of healthcare are much more negative in terms of standards of care (Patients Association, 2015), suggesting that best evidence needs to also translate into understanding the subjective experience of care. This is because nursing practice is reliant on the subjective understanding of the person undertaking the practice as well as their interpretations of the evidence their practice is based upon; it is often this piece of the knowledge jigsaw which nurses attain through reflection.

Implementing best evidence through technological processes can sometimes lead to intimacy becoming lost, reducing opportunities for subjective assessment of patients and developing the *professional craft* knowledge so important to making subjective sense of evidence.

Different types of subjectivities start to emerge from the complexity of people's lives. The cultural subject emerges from expressions of beliefs, values and group norms (Jarvis, 2006). What kind of student nurse you are and how you think is defined in part by your biography, but also through existing as a student nurse in the professional world of nursing. Similarly, patients will be defined by their own histories and cultures, but also through the experience of being a patient in the context of the care setting.

These can all be influential on the care experience. People are *knowledgeable agents* interpreting their existence (Giddens, cited in Delanty and Strydom, 2003, p378). Therefore, any interpretations people apply to their experience will by their very nature be unique and consequently difficult to explain to others. Observed behaviours do not tell the whole story as people adapt what they are doing moment by moment in response to how they interpret their world, which is subjective. The **Hawthorne effect** – where behaviours change because people know they are being observed – is one example of the limitations that may arise with evidence that claims to be objective but ignores the importance of relationships and interaction between people (Barker, 2010). A subjective account is more revealing because of 'insider knowledge' than an account by someone trying to interpret or translate that experience into a more generalisable form (West et al., 2007). What this suggests is that practitioners need to consider how sufficient their insight of patient experience is and what this is based upon. You may want to work through the following scenario to help you to understand the difference between insider knowledge and that of someone trying to understand their experience from the outside.

Activity 5.1 — *Critical thinking*

Brigid was a lady in her 30s who worked in an office. Four years ago she had noticed a loss of sensation in her right leg that made walking cumbersome at times. This persisted for three weeks and then went away. It recurred in her other leg a year later and again lasted for only a few weeks. Brigid noticed that she was also tired during these episodes. Her doctor could find little wrong and assumed Brigid was stressed.

Brigid knew her own body and still had a nagging sense that something was wrong. She did not think that work was particularly stressful at the times the loss of sensation occurred. She noted that the loss of sensation also varied in intensity, becoming worse when she had a bath. Brigid felt that her doctor did not believe her and this made it harder for her to catalogue and report her symptoms accurately.

How might you help to make sense of Brigid's experience?

There is an outline answer to this question at the end of the chapter.

Patients have a better understanding of what an illness or disease process feels like than the healthcare practitioners who look after them – we can only measure the signs of disease, but need patients to tell us what the symptoms are. The nature of health knowledge is not exclusive to professionals (Pattison, 2001); while professionals may have a developed understanding of the objective nature of illness and injury, it is the person experiencing the issue who is the expert in how they are affected. It is important that nurses try to employ methods that can tap into this patient understanding in order to identify how their interventions might be experienced by patients.

Objective data can provide information about physiological responses, but how a person experiences their body and changes within it will always be subjective. Through sharing practice issues and reflecting on their practice – as explained in the book *Reflective Practice in Nursing* in this series – practitioners are able to advance their practice knowledge in subjective ways that interrogate and analyse what knowledge is based upon and how others interpret it.

Reflexivity, based on reflecting on their subjective insights, is how nurses can critically explore the organisations and structures within which they exist and consider what influence they might have to change their situation or be changed by it (Merrill and West, 2009). The critically **reflexive** practitioner utilises various strategies for developing knowledge (Brookfield, 2005); these include engaging with their historical experience, reading and understanding literature, and reflecting on practice and social interaction. Literature can set the experience within a body of knowledge that might include research studies as well as other practitioner accounts that are instrumental in validating experience. Being reflexive involves focusing on opportunities for learning by interrogating subjective perceptions, and considering issues of power and how people are thought of or spoken about.

Critical reflexivity means considering what is being asked and how this might translate into personal practice and how this relates to the evidence available in different forms. This reflexive stance offers an opportunity to examine our assumptions and how we might be implicated in the structures we create in everyday working (Bolton, 2014). Making sense of subjective experience involves understanding how this has evolved over time, how it fits with the experiences of others, what the study of experiences has revealed and what actually happens in practice.

Healthcare is constantly changing, and as nurses we are faced with new knowledge every day. Responding reflexively to changes in knowledge involves being open to experience and re-evaluating what might have been viewed as *fixed bodies of knowledge* (West et al., 2007, p18) – in other words, appraising the evidence of what knowledge already exists and why it might need to change and examining its relevance and potential effectiveness for our practice and how we might use it. This strongly reflects many of the dispositions and influences on practice identified in Figure 1.1 on p21, which you may like to revisit in order to help contextualise the current discussion.

Such reflexive consideration may lead to new insights into assumptions about how knowledge is used and how practitioners may be instrumental in developing evidence through their reworking of knowledge. Reflexive evaluation is an important method for transforming personal viewpoints in positive ways (Cangelosi, 2008).

If experience is founded on rigorously tested knowledge, then it might be argued that intuition will also be research-based because the resulting knowledge derives from applying research evidence to practice through the mediums of reflection and reflexivity. For example, when thinking about handwashing there is a wealth of research evidence that identifies best practice for completing this, but until subjective sense is made of the actions and steps, the process will not be embedded into regular practice, or possibly even be adhered to. There are factors that may intervene – for example, physical states such as skin allergies and psychological factors such as resistance and stress (Elliott, 2009). In order for practice to become evidence-based, it is necessary to first make subjective sense of evidence by being reflexive. Completing Activity 5.2 might help you to identify how to develop some critical reflexivity.

Activity 5.2   *Critical thinking*

Think about what you know about nutritional care by considering the following questions.

- What do you know about handwashing?
- How have you developed this knowledge?
- Has this knowledge changed at all and if so how?
- How important is it to you to keep this knowledge updated?
- What might you do about updating your knowledge?
- What might prevent you from updating your knowledge?
- What might be the consequences of updating/not updating your knowledge, to the patient, to you, to the profession, to the organisation?
- How does updating your knowledge alter what you do in practice?

There is an outline answer to this activity at the end of the chapter.

Relating subjective experience to other forms of evidence

Subjectivity may be constrained into a more acceptable form by dominating factors such as policy and procedures (West et al., 2007). Underpinning the drive for modernisation of the health service is the commitment to improving quality, and evidence-based practice is viewed as one way to help achieve this (Craig and Smyth, 2007). In this way it becomes possible to identify what decisions are based upon and their potential outcomes. Qualitative research aims to find contextual and personal explanations for phenomena, while quantitative research aims to measure and record instances and events. Nevertheless, quantifying reality alone can miss cues that help to extend the understanding of events, particularly from the patient's perspective. Such aspects may include attitudes, beliefs, thinking and feeling. Who, why, where and when are the questions of the qualitative thinker (Janesick, 2003) and can be seen to link to those of critical reflexivity as detailed earlier. Asking how people are feeling is also important to help understand effects. Such questioning is essential to ensure that you are always challenging your own practice and relating to the evidence available for what you are doing.

Some forms of research try to categorise and predict what sometimes might be more confused and subjective. For example, it may be possible to predict how a person is likely to react to a particular medication, but how that medication makes someone feel is likely to vary from person to person and may influence their compliance with a treatment regimen, which will ultimately impact its effectiveness. In nursing, we are dealing with human beings, each of whom is unique; this makes consideration of subjective experience important. Illness is a **phenomenological** experience (Carel, 2008). For example, feeling pain is a very subjective experience, and although pain assessment tools may be able to categorise levels, the actual intensity of the experience remains something very personal (Buswell, 1998). Undertaking Activity 5.3 might help you to consider ways in which understanding the client perspective might be important and relevant to your practice.

Activity 5.3 *Reflection*

Think about how pain is measured in your present or recent placement. What evidence supports this measurement? Now think about what prompts you to administer pain medication. Now think about a time when you experienced significant pain. Was there any alteration to the way you approached patients in practice following your subjective experience and if so, how?

There is an outline answer to this activity at the end of the chapter.

How we react as individual nurses to different situations is relevant to the learning that we take from those experiences. In some mainstream research traditions people are viewed as cognitive information-processing subjects, missing the more intimate and diverse factors of learning such as the emotional and biographical (West et al., 2007). What this means is that people may focus on functional understanding and consequently miss subjective knowledge that is part of the lived embodied experience from which processes and interactions arise. Nevertheless, there is also a danger in assuming that subjective experience and acting on intuitive knowing is enough. It is likely that you will have come across the expressions 'We have always done things this way' or 'I know from experience'. The danger with this is that it is someone else's experience; your interpretation or level of experience may not be identical to theirs and therefore the results of your actions may not be identical either. There are other issues with relying too heavily on subjective experience which include misinterpretation and misunderstanding of a situation.

Concept summary: problems of subjective experience

We all know someone who has lived into their eighties while smoking 20 cigarettes a day. To some subjective observers this suggests that there is no impact of smoking on the longevity of life, but we know this is not true and that in fact a smoker who died in their eighties may well have made it to their nineties or beyond had they never smoked.

Many patients want antibiotics from their GP when they have a cold because in the past they have had antibiotics when they had a cold and have got better; they therefore assume it is the antibiotics which have cured them. What we know in fact is that they would have got better anyway regardless of the antibiotics because most colds are viral and antibiotics have no effect on viral diseases.

A range of evidence is required in order to choose the most appropriate action for the circumstances. Hamm's cognitive continuum (cited in Thompson and Dowding, 2002, p13) suggests that intuition and scientific knowledge are at different ends of a spectrum of evidence where judgements are formed using different thought processes (see also Standing, 2011). Analytical modes use research and experimental evidence from which to draw inferences while peer discussion invites the experience of others to help inform judgements, and the intuitive mode is based on developed expertise. However, in practice a number of these modes may be in use at the same time within a given situation and, therefore, categorising different forms of evidence in a hierarchy may have limitations. For example, empirical research informs choices in wound management but subjective experience also directs action. Consider the following scenario to help you to identify how subjective experience relates to different forms of evidence.

Activity 5.4   *Critical thinking*

Gerald is a man in his eighties who has diabetes. He is admitted to hospital with a urinary tract infection that has made him confused. What evidence will be used to manage Gerald's care?

There is an outline answer to this question at the end of the chapter.

Working through the scenario you may have identified that the kind of evidence used for practice also relates to different stances that might be adopted.

Particular stances

Evidence-based practice focuses on the need for research awareness in order to provide good-quality patient care. Thinking about the evidence on which to base your practice requires effort to interrogate the appropriateness of that evidence for the situation. Part of such interrogation involves considering the stance of the evidence and whether it also relates to a medical or nursing model of care. For example, a medical model has tended to employ a **reductionist**, rational approach to finding solutions to medical problems by concentrating on signs and symptoms that enable the calculation of risk and benefit, and a generalised response to intervention (Greenhalgh, 2010). In this stance health is viewed from a deficit perspective with problems becoming deconstructed in order to identify potential solutions. Taking such a stance encourages objective decision-making, which is an important part of being a professional, but it can also become detached from your and the patient's subjective experience, affecting the quality of therapeutic relationships. A narrative approach considers the whole story of a problem. Reading the following case study may help to illustrate this point.

Case study: The onset of the menopause

Damaris was in her late fifties and had become increasingly withdrawn. Her husband was very worried and finally managed to get her to see their GP, John. At the appointment John could get hardly any response from Damaris and was reliant on her husband Kosta's narrative of what had

---

continued ...

been happening. John arranged a blood test and prescribed an anti-depressant. Damaris refused to take the medication and eventually refused to eat as well. John saw her again and arranged a psychiatric referral as the blood test had not revealed any problems. At the mental health unit Damaris and Kosta were met by Gemma, a mental health nurse. Gemma spoke to them both while they waited. Damaris was eventually seen by Sara, the psychiatrist. Sara asked Damaris how she was feeling and if anything had changed. Damaris spoke haltingly with Kosta filling in gaps in her narration. From this narration Sara was able to establish a picture of Damaris's increasingly depressive feelings as her children had left home. She also determined that Damaris was experiencing hot flushes and mood swings. Sara asked Gemma to take another blood test to measure Damaris's hormone levels. Sara asked Damaris to come back to see her again when the results were available. Gemma talked gently to Damaris while taking the blood sample. Damaris began to relax. Gemma used this opportunity to give her some nutritional advice on foods that could be helpful during the menopause. Damaris left the unit feeling that she had been listened to. When she arrived home she managed to eat a little supper.

The case study may have helped you to understand that while the evidence on which diagnosis and treatments are based needs to be rigorous, there also needs to be some interaction and attachment to the person to help them to make sense of the implications for their lives and to be able to work with the information (you will recall we said that we can see and measure signs of disease, but people experiencing ill health have to tell us about the symptoms). Barriers to implementing evidence-based practice include problems with understanding the research findings and being able to translate them into practice in a way that is acceptable to the practitioner and patient (Brown, 1995). Inclusion of consideration of subjective experience can promote human elements that are important to feeling cared for and for your learning.

Organisational models

Organisational models use deductive and inductive approaches to promote adoption and implementation of evidence-based practice (Kitson et al., 1996). The deductive process involves audit and drafting clinical guidelines from rigorously tested knowledge. The inductive process entails observing, interpreting and analysing daily occurrences generating new theory. These methods are useful for formulating policies (Couchman and Dawson, 1995). Policies and procedures can help to legitimate nurses' knowledge (Manias and Street, 2000).

Policies are agreed courses of action that have been endorsed by the organisation, such as clinical protocols or guidelines detailing mandatory or recommended approaches to treating specific clinical problems. Standards provide statements of good practice with benchmarks against which practice can be audited. However, overreliance on an organisational stance that describes what should be done in particular circumstances can also result in formulaic judgements and difficulty when faced with situations that require flexibility. As experience is produced from practice every day it would seem that it also plays some part in generating the evidence base. By undertaking Activity 5.5 you will be able to understand how policies are formed.

Activity 5.5   *Research and finding out*

When you are next in your placement, look at the policy folders or intranet and choose a policy to examine. Consider the following.

- What category does the policy fall into in terms of protocol or guideline?
- Is the reason for the policy explained?
- Is the document evidence-based and referenced?
- Does the document reflect best practice by identifying procedures to be followed?
- Is the policy written in a clear and jargon-free style?

There is an outline answer to this activity at the end of the chapter.

Action research

Action research is another inductive process through which practice may be moved forward and involves reflection on practice and description of change potential and problems. The outcomes and claims to knowledge of action research as a methodology are still hotly debated (Kemmis and McTaggert, 2008). You can read more about this in the final chapter of the companion book in this series on *Understanding Research for Nursing Students* (Ellis, 2016).

The **gestalt** moment where understanding comes together is an integral part of this type of evidence that enables the practitioner to make such connections for their own learning (McNiff and Whitehead, 2002). The focus within this stance is on the practitioner's learning. A number of philosophies can inform this approach, including the scientific perspective, interpreting patterns and behaviours, and removing barriers and constraints to enable individuals to change. There are fine lines between routine problem solving, reviewing practice and interrogating practice to develop an evidence base. The nature of knowledge is that it grows, at least in part, from a fusing of objective experience with subjective understanding. Gadamer (1989) describes this as a fusing of horizons from the perspective of the investigator who brings their own preconceptions (current knowledge) to a situation to develop new understandings. McNiff and Whitehead (2002) suggest that it is important to 'organically' grow theory within practice. However, this assumes that practice is the measure of the validity of nursing knowledge.

Both nursing practice and nursing theory are important. Practice without theory may lack direction and could be dangerous, while theory without practice becomes pointless because it remains abstract. Action research develops understanding of real-life issues and ways of dealing with them (Williamson et al., 2012). Undertaking the following activity can help you to identify how practice might produce theory.

Activity 5.6   *Reflection*

Think about what you have learnt from your practice so far. How might you frame this process to look more rigorously at the evidence base of your practice?

There is an outline answer to this activity at the end of the chapter.

Making sense of your practice means also contextualising the lived experience of the practitioner and the patient being cared for.

Contextualising lived experience

It is important to be able to integrate theory with the lived experience of practice in order to be able to focus upon what evidence is needed and how it is used. Making sense of the evidence base from different stances is likely to be achieved through engagement with intellectual activities to support creativity in nursing practice, and development and innovation.

Fasnacht (2003, p196) claims that nursing's interpretation of creativity is expressed in terms of the 'product' rather than the 'processes'. The product referred to here is that of nursing outcomes as opposed to the process of the nursing care. However, it could be suggested that it is necessary to have a goal in order to develop a process that enables you to reach it. Making sense of subjective experience is part of this process. It could be contended that without an understanding of patient experiences and concerns (as they are the end users of healthcare), education and practice remain sterile and unrelated, and the evidence base for practice is harder to grasp. As patient care crosses many professional boundaries, these experiences are better considered holistically, rather than examined as fragments that may omit important professional insight.

Experience is produced from practice and records the outcome of that practice. Contextualising and making sense of subjective experience involves thinking about the human factors inherent in practice and how these might be influential to and influenced by different forms of enquiry. The process is illustrated in Figure 5.1.

Constantly reflecting on our practice and evaluating processes that are successful and those that are less so will help alert us to how our practice is evolving. Methods that can add rigour to processes of reflection and evaluation are clinical supervision and critical reflection as explained in the book *Reflective Practice in Nursing* in this series. Such evaluation involves comparing the evidence of successful interaction and intervention with alternatives, to help plan future actions that are likely to be effective.

Clinical supervision involves the guidance of an experienced facilitator to add depth to the reflection undertaken by the practitioner. This might occur within practice or the university, in groups or individually. It is also possible to develop a form of peer supervision that involves peer questioning of subjective experiences, interpretations and the actions, decisions and knowledge

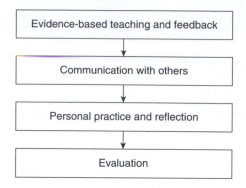

Figure 5.1: The process of understanding the context of evidence

used to underpin these. However, the rigour of this is likely to be limited by the level of knowledge of that peer and therefore this form of supervision may be more useful to develop some of the questions that you might want to ask yourself.

Making sense of subjective experience also requires evaluating what you read and are told, and how this fits with practice and research findings. Maintaining a reflective log that you discuss regularly with your tutor is another way in which you can contextualise your lived experience within the framework of evidence-based teaching. Used together, these methods could offer a supported reflexivity that can help to integrate subjective knowledge, practice and theory. Undertaking Activity 5.7 might help you to develop some strategies for contextualising and evaluating your subjective experience.

Activity 5.7   *Reflection*

Use the following questions to interrogate your subjective experience:

- What is informing my knowledge and practice?
- How do I feel about this?
- What works well/less well and why might this be?
- What might need to change and how will I do this?
- What am I taking forward?
- What have I learnt from this?

As this activity is based on your experiences, there is no outline answer at the end of the chapter.

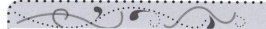

Chapter summary

This chapter has considered how subjective experience is relevant and might be used both to create evidence for practice and to create a context for other different forms of evidence that may be used for practice. In particular, the role of subjective experience in

continued ... •••

> supporting learning about practice and accessing the patient/client experience as part of identifying the effectiveness of practice has been explored. Different stances may be employed but ultimately practice deals with unique human beings and therefore human factors need to be included. Utilising a holistic approach that is inclusive of different forms of enquiry, evidence and stances will enrich your knowledge and practice within the ethos of nursing.

Activities: Brief outline answers

Activity 5.1: Critical thinking (page 83)

Making sense of Brigid's symptoms requires *listening* to her experience. This means attending not only to the physiological effects but also to how she *feels* within her own body. Doing this helps to access the insider knowledge that external measurement may miss. You could help Brigid by talking to her and documenting her experience. This can record whether there is a pattern to her symptoms – or particular triggers – and so start to establish evidence based on her subjective experience.

Activity 5.2: Critical thinking (page 85)

Nutritional care has changed over time.

- Your knowledge about handwashing may include understanding how to wash your hands and when. You may consider the water temperature, the washing agents you use and whether you subsequently use an alcohol rub.
- It is likely that you will have developed this knowledge through integrating theory from classes at university and reading with what you have observed in practice. You may have observed a variety of practice, some of which may not correspond with what you have read/been taught. It is at this point that you would need to identify what is the most appropriate practice through reflecting on the evidence base of what you know.
- Your knowledge is likely to have started from the fixed point of the theory you were taught at university. It is likely to have progressed and expanded as your practice has included a variety of patients and clients, allowing you to make subjective sense of the theory by putting it into practice. Equally, new research findings are likely to become incorporated into teaching and organisational guidance, and therefore inform your thinking as you progress through the programme.
- How important it is to you to keep this knowledge updated will depend on your subjective interpretations of being a nurse.
- To keep your knowledge up to date you might read journal articles regularly (see Chapter 2 for strategies for identifying sources of appropriate literature) and discuss practice with peers and practice colleagues. You might even be involved in an action learning set or clinical supervision group who could help you with this.
- What might prevent you from updating your knowledge is likely to include lack of time, tiredness, not knowing how to update your knowledge and maybe even a lack of desire to do so, thinking that others know best.
- The consequences of updating your knowledge could be: for the patient, that they do not receive potentially dangerous care; for you, that you increase your knowledge and understanding; for the profession, that you are upholding the reputation of the profession; and for the organisation, that it is seen to be facilitating good care and preventing the spread of infection. The consequences of not updating your knowledge and practice might be: for the patient, that they develop an infection because of poor hygiene practice; for you, that you fail to keep your understanding up to date; for the profession, that nurses are viewed as ineffective; for the organisation, that standards of care are poor.

- You may notice that as you receive ongoing training and development about hand hygiene that your practice of handwashing improves and that how you wash becomes more intuitive than something you think about regularly.

Activity 5.3: Reflection (page 86)

It is likely that some kind of pain assessment tool is utilised in the practice area. This will be associated with a range of medication and a formula for administration. These are likely to be based on the findings of research studies. However, you are also likely to take note of patient body language and expressions of pain to help guide your assessment of the need for pain relief. If you have experienced significant pain yourself, your awareness of the difference in feeling and experience is likely to be heightened. This may develop your alertness to the variety of pain intensity and subtle signs, and to what questions to ask to help the patient to access the appropriate medication at the appropriate time.

Activity 5.4: Critical thinking (page 87)

You may have identified the type of urinary infection Gerald had from sending a urine sample for scientific evaluation. You are likely to have used physiological data, such as measuring his oxygen saturation level, to check whether his confusion was caused by hypoxia. You will have interacted with Gerald to find out how he was feeling. You may have checked research findings for the most suitable antibiotic treatment and latest guidance on other measures, such as fluid intake advice, to alleviate symptoms and support recovery. Throughout this you might have been reviewing your own experience of what you are observing of Gerald's illness and response to treatment and how your knowledge is developing. Crucially you will also interact with Gerald's family to ascertain whether his confusion was in fact normal for him.

Activity 5.5: Research and finding out (page 89)

Policies should be complete, yet simple and easy to read for a potentially diverse audience. Policies fall into two categories: clinical and administrative. You may have identified that the information can be divided into three levels: actual policy, applicable procedures and necessary instructions. In terms of evidence the policy is likely to have:

- identified the problem and described the regulatory background and expected benefits;
- described the chronological series of interrelated steps to comply with the policy;
- distinguished who the policy relates to;
- determined related information such as underpinning references and training required;
- identified which parts of the organisation, or which personnel, if any, are excluded;
- identified where specific questions can be referred to.

Activity 5.6: Reflection (page 90)

Practice development needs to be patient rather than institutionally focused in order to effectively address patient care. Therefore, the process might focus on the following areas:

- defining why change is needed and what is desired;
- appraising the evidence that supports or refutes the proposed change;
- identifying achievable and evidence-based change;
- identifying key components of your development and their fit with current practices;
- determining what support structures, outcomes and resources are required;
- planning how your development will be implemented and evaluated.

Further reading

Carel, H (2008) *Illness*. Stocksfield: Acumen.

This book will help you to understand how important the subjective view is to understanding and listening to patients as a basis for practice.

Higgs, J, Richardson, B and Abrandt Dahlgren, M (eds) (2004) *Developing practice knowledge for health professionals.* Edinburgh: Butterworth Heinemann.

This book will help you to understand how different kinds of knowledge relate and are relevant to the practice of nursing.

Jarvis, P (1999) *The practitioner-researcher: developing theory from practice.* San Francisco, CA: Jossey-Bass/Wiley.

Reading this book will help you to develop an understanding of how evidence can emerge from practice to inform theory.

Useful website

www.evidence.nhs-uk This website is useful for finding information on clinical topics and guidelines.

Chapter 6
Collaborative working to achieve evidence-based care

Peter Ellis

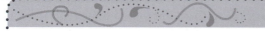

continued ...

9. People can trust the newly registered graduate nurse to treat them as partners and work with them to make a holistic and systematic assessment of their needs; to develop a personalised plan that is based on mutual understanding and respect for their individual situation, promoting health and well-being, minimising risk of harm and promoting their safety at all times.

12. People can trust the newly registered graduate nurse to respond to their feedback and a wide range of other sources to learn, develop and improve services.

13. People can trust the newly registered graduate nurse to promote continuity when their care is to be transferred to another service or person.

Chapter aims

After reading this chapter, you will be able to:

- demonstrate awareness as to why working with others in the planning of evidence-based care is important;
- identify the different groups of individuals it is important to work with to achieve evidenced care;
- understand some of the barriers to interprofessional evidence-based care delivery;
- be able to describe why service users' views are important in the delivery of evidence-based nursing practice.

Introduction

So far in this book we have explored some of the skills you need to work as an individual nurse providing evidence-based nursing care. We have identified some challenges that might face the nurse who is attempting to provide evidence-based care and have presented some tools for you to take on board for yourself when developing as an evidential nurse who is ready for the challenges of lifelong learning.

Nursing care does not take place in a vacuum. The complexities of modern care mean that there is a need for any number of professional and voluntary care givers to provide the care that any individual patient needs. There are also care delivery issues that need to be accounted for, such as the experience of care and the individual needs and wishes of each patient.

This chapter will present an overview of some of the issues that face nurses when working with others, including patients. It will also present an argument that working effectively with others is an important element in the delivery of evidence-based nursing care. As in the rest of the book, the issues here are that no single element of care can be considered on its own and that one element of the caring process does not take precedence over another. Rather, the argument about evidence-based care presented in this book frames evidence-based nursing as the delivery of holistic, multifaceted and multiprofessional care, which is supported by lifelong learning, ethical sensitivity and moral activity, reflection and reflexivity as well as an understanding of research, experiential elements of learning and, above all, the needs and wishes of the individual patient.

It is plain to see that the argument made here is quite complex. It is an argument that responds to some of the greyness existing at the boundaries of theory and practice, and, it is hoped, prepares or further develops the ability of nurses to advance the quality of their practice in a meaningful, well-thought-out and patient-focused manner.

This chapter illuminates some of the elements of Figure 1.1 ('The influences on and dispositions of an evidence-based nurse'; see p21) in which we saw delivering patient-centred care requires multiple strands of conscious decision-making to run simultaneously. We saw how various dispositions (or elements of our character) affect the ways in which we can engage as evidential, patient-centred practitioners. One of these dispositions is to be 'other regarding'.

Furthermore, we saw in the 'influences on practice' that there is a role for 'patient preference' as well as the 'views of other professionals'. What they amount to is the need to manage personal choices and behaviours, as well as seeking and nurturing interpersonal relationships, which, with resolve and some practice, enable nurses to deliver care in a manner that is both evidence-driven and patient-centred. This chapter is about exploring the interpersonal relationship aspect of this evidence-based nursing practice.

Service users' views

Taking account of the views of services users, the patient's voice, is high on the governmental agenda (DH, 2000, 2010). This agenda is clearly reflected in the standards for competence and essential skill clusters required of nurses by the Nursing and Midwifery Council (NMC, 2010), some of which are highlighted at the start of the chapter.

What, then, is a service user? Service users fall into one of two categories: those who are current users of caring services such as health and social care, and those who are potential future users of these same services. This explains why the term 'patient' is not used consistently throughout this chapter. In fact, we are all actual and potential users of health and social care (Connelly and Seden, 2003) but most of the time we are not patients and would not necessarily like to be thought of as such. Most of us have accessed care on a number of occasions in our lives, be that because we are ill or because we are being screened for disease or vaccinated against some communicable disease.

What, then, is important about the views of services users about the delivery of care? Clearly, most service users have a limited amount of knowledge about the hard science of care delivery and may not have a view about the quality of X-ray services, the choice of wound dressing used in the hospital or the biochemistry services' use of particular assays. What they – and we – do have, however, is significant experience of how we like to be treated in the care environment, and how we experience both illness and care. We all also have our own views about the extent of the care that we may wish to receive and how this affects us as individuals.

> ## Activity 6.1   *Reflection*
>
> Think back to a time when you, or a friend or relative, were the recipient of hospital care. What sorts of things served to make your use of the services more pleasant and what things did you think were not so good?
>
> *As this activity is based on your own reflection, there is no outline answer at the end of the chapter.*

Clearly, as well as the human elements of taking account of people's views about their own care, there are several moral and ethical imperatives that we, as nurses, must take account of in the delivery of care (Ellis, 2014). Perhaps the most important ethical principle, as it applies to this section of the book, is the imperative to respect the autonomy of individuals.

Autonomy is about the freedom to choose. In part the process of consent supports this freedom of choice and involves the nurse who is delivering care in ensuring that the recipient of care understands what is going to happen to them (information giving and individual competence), is free from coercion (undue pressure) and understands what the alternative forms of care are – if there are any (Beauchamp and Childress, 2013).

Issues of both advocacy and empowerment are important to the evidence-based nurse who is focused on delivering high-quality care that is based on evaluated knowledge and is what the patient actually wants. Some definitions regard advocacy as simply the process of representing the views of someone to someone else; for example, Dubler (1992, p85) defines advocacy within the caring professions as *acting to the limit of professional ability to provide for the client's interests and needs as the patient defines them.* In Dubler's view, then, an advocate puts to one side their own view of a situation and represents only the point of view of the person they are advocating for. This view of advocacy actually represents the true meaning of the word quite well as it stresses the importance of only representing the views of the client and no one else. This simple view of advocacy falls a little short of the realities of nursing care, though, in that it makes assumptions about the capacity (mental competence) and understanding of the facts by the individual client. It also misses the point where the decision is tainted by misapprehension or negative prior experiences.

Within this book, advocacy as it applies to the evidence-based nurse is a term used to define a process of representing the views of a service user when the nurse has ensured that they have discussed the nature of the intervention with the service user and have highlighted the alternatives available and the evidence for each potential course of action. Furthermore, the morally active evidence-based nurse will also ensure that the service user has understood what has been said and that they are able and free to make a rational choice about what they want to happen.

Empowerment and advocacy in this respect are seen as different stages along the same continuum of patient-focused care, with empowerment defined as enabling service users to speak for themselves about what choices they have made about their care (Nolan and Ellis, 2008). As in the definition of advocacy, the service user must be in receipt of the information they need to make their decision and they must understand the information. This definition of empowerment, like that of advocacy, recognises that the majority of people are able and willing to engage in decision-making about their own care. Both definitions further recognise that this is the patient's right and that some people will choose to exercise it and others will not or, indeed, cannot.

Activity 6.2   *Reflection*

Return to the model of evidence-based nursing presented in Chapter 1 (see Figure 1.1 on p21) and reflect on the nature of the process of decision-making discussed there. Identify especially the ethical elements of the model and the elements that apply to decision-making that take into account patient preferences and the dispositions of the evidence-based nurse that are 'other regarding'. How do you see these as contributing to user consultation as highlighted in this section?

An outline answer is provided at the end of the chapter.

Service users' views also extend to understanding the views of individuals – and groups of individuals – who are not currently in receipt of care. These views help to shape our understanding of the context within which care is received and therefore how it might best be delivered.

On a macro level these views are sought through governmental and local authority consultation while more disease-specific groups might be a source of understanding and knowledge about specific elements of care services delivery. In her report on privacy and dignity in hospitals, the Chief Nursing Officer for Great Britain reported on consultations with over 2000 patients who viewed the cleanliness of hospitals as their number one priority, with issues such as 'having information' and 'thoughtful staff' also high on their list of priorities (DH, 2007). The Cancer Partnership Project – a joint venture between Macmillan Cancer Relief and the Department of Health that consulted widely among professionals and cancer sufferers on the provision and delivery of cancer services – was regarded as a successful model of consultation and led to effective changes in cancer care provision in the UK (Sitzia et al., 2004).

More locally, patient groups, such as hospital-affiliated kidney or cardiac patients' associations, play a useful role in identifying areas of concern for patients and care providers as well as in supporting changes to care delivery.

What is evident is that a move away from professional-driven care has occurred in the UK and that the voice of patients is increasingly being heard.

Activity 6.3   *Communication*

Next time you are in practice, spend some time talking to some patients about their experience of the care that they are receiving. Make quite sure they understand that it is their experience of their care that you are interested in; this means what it feels like for them, how it affects their lives and families and not the technicalities of the disease. Ensure when you ask the patient to discuss their experiences that they understand there will be no adverse effects on their care as a result of their discussion with you. Reflect on what they are telling you about the care that they are receiving and compare this to the answers you gave for Activity 6.1.

As this activity is based on your own reflection, there is no outline answer at the end of the chapter.

Evidence operates at two levels. At the first level it provides evidence for care in its own right. That is to say, the experience of the patient, the *symptoms* they express and their interpretation of the care they receive provide evidence for nursing. For example, only the patient can know if they feel pain, are upset or anxious – remember as nurses we cannot directly measure symptoms, we can only see and measure signs of illness and disease. We cannot validate these symptoms through direct objective mechanisms as we have no machine to measure pain or anxiety as such. We can, however, use some objective measures to validate what they are telling us, such as noting a rise in blood pressure or that the patient is sweating, crying or perhaps trembling. We can also validate what the patient is telling us about what they feel through our own subjective interpretation and understanding of what they are experiencing on a human level – through common understanding of human experience, what might be called **intersubjectivity**.

At the second level, subjective evidence might serve to validate observations that we have made for ourselves using more objective measures. For example, if we take a blood sugar reading for a patient with diabetes and find that they are hypoglycemic (have a low blood sugar level), we might expect them to tell us they feel tired, hungry or confused.

What these examples show is that in our day-to-day practice we see interplay between what we can measure and observe for ourselves and what the patient tells us. The argument here is that whichever way round the information comes to us – patients telling us their symptoms or us observing signs – as nurses we are often alert to and able to handle the interplay between more than one source of evidence for practice at any one time. In *Understanding Research for Nursing Students* (also in this series), Chapter 6 discusses in detail the concept of triangulation which is about validating information using more than one information source.

Sometimes evidence can be contradictory: the patient tells us they are not in pain but we observe them wincing or gritting their teeth. On such occasions it is communication that helps us to express our concerns to the patient and demonstrate both our disposition to be 'other regarding' and the advancing influence of increasing 'practice knowledge' (see Figure 1.1 on p21). Evidently, in this scenario there is also a need to exercise the disposition of being both 'ethically sensitive' and 'morally active' in seeking via good communication to act in what will be in the best interests of our patient.

What seems clear is that whatever we think about the motivations behind the advance of the evidence-based practice agenda, as nurses we practise it daily within our working lives. Perhaps awaking our understanding of what evidence-based practice means for nursing on a more macro scale requires we become more aware of how the principles of evidence-based nursing practice operate at this micro level to inform our day-to-day practice.

In this section we have identified that user consultation is an important element of the government's agenda and that it is identified by the NMC as a required competency for all nurses. We have seen there is a moral imperative for the evidence-based nurse to take into account service users' views, and that advocacy and empowerment are key strategies for making this a reality of the care process. We have also seen how interaction and exploration of subjectivity enable the nurse operating on a day-to-day basis to be evidence-based in their care provision and that understanding how this operates might help us to understand the importance of evidence-based practice for nursing on a much broader scale.

Before we go on to explore further strategies for identifying service users' views, it is important that we identify some of the barriers to consultation that might impact on the evidence-based nurse.

Barriers to patient consultation

By understanding the potential problems we are better able to understand how something might be made to work better. We have identified that user consultation takes place at two key levels: at the one-to-one level, where the concern is the care of an individual; and at the group level, where the concern is the general care provided to a group of patients. We will examine some of the barriers to effective consultation at each of these levels.

Communication and interaction with patients are the cornerstone of good nursing care. Communication is time-consuming, however, and the sharing of information and ensuring that information is understood can take precious time out of the nurse's day. Information and frank and open discussion are not easy to undertake in the ward environment where there are distractions and the very real possibility that a consultation will be overheard by others. Our own lack of knowledge and a fear of demonstrating this to patients may make some nurses feel uncomfortable about discussing options for care.

As well as physical and personal barriers to communication and consultation, there are barriers that are created because of the position we hold, or feel we hold, in the multidisciplinary team. This may lead some nurses to be coy about discussing possibilities of care with patients because they feel that ultimately someone else will make the decision about care. At other times we may feel unable to put into language that the patient will understand the various options for their care. We may feel we are best placed to make a decision about the care of patients, especially where individual patients appear less than able to make such decisions for themselves – as might be the case for some adults with learning difficulties.

It is situations like these that highlight the very real need for morality and ethics to feature strongly in any framework of evidence-based nursing. It would be easier to operate in a moral vacuum where we make choices for our patients based on what we think are in their medical (or nursing) best interests (Benjamin and Curtis, 1992). However, such an understanding of evidence-based care misses the point that 'best interests' not only include physical elements but also psychosocial, and perhaps even spiritual, aspects of who we are as human beings (Dworkin, 1993). This highlights the need not only for a subjective and intersubjective interpretation of evidence, but also for good communication and a commitment to morally active nursing, advocacy and empowerment.

Patients themselves may present a number of difficulties for the nurse trying to discuss care options. The vulnerability that may arise out of illness, physical or mental disability, age or language can stand in the way of effective two-way communication.

Activity 6.4   *Reflection*

Think about the last time you had to share difficult information with a patient or family member. What was going on in your mind as you talked to them and how did their response to you make you feel? Were you surprised at their response? How did you manage to find the right words to say and how did you know you had said the right things?

As this activity is based on your own reflection, there is no outline answer at the end of the chapter.

Other barriers to good communication and taking account of the opinions and experiences of patients include our own orientations to other people and the beliefs we hold about the value of this sort of interaction. Sometimes we make assumptions about what patients do and do not know because they are not care professionals like us or, indeed, because they come from a caring background and therefore we feel they should know about their own care needs. At other times we make the assumption that because they have been seen by another member of the team they have all of the information they need and we do not need to engage with them because they do not need to hear the information twice or because it is hard for us to have difficult conversations.

On many occasions, we feel too self-conscious to explore the patient's opinions about their care because their condition is too embarrassing to talk about or we feel out of our depth discussing issues such as death or mental illness. Sometimes the patients' wishes, opinions and experiences take us out of our comfort zones.

So how might we function in such scenarios and how might we develop the characteristics and dispositions of the morally active evidence-based nurse?

Working effectively with service users

In order to overcome the difficulties and barriers that stop us communicating well with patients, we have to take the initiative. It is not really possible to be an ethically sensitive or morally active evidence-based nurse without communicating with patients about their experiences and engaging them in the planning of their own care. At a one-to-one level there are a number of strategies we can employ that will make this role easier and allow us to add being 'other regarding' and 'engaged with self' to our list of personal qualities.

Overcoming barriers to communication as a student or junior nurse requires us to make time to spend constructively with our patients, and to use this time wisely. Clearly, the personal barriers to communication are ours to overcome. Investing time in reflection, either singly or in a group, is a useful strategy in allowing us to identify these barriers and ways in which they might be overcome (Jasper, 2003). Some strategies towards achieving good communication are presented in Table 6.1.

Table 6.1: Some strategies for achieving good communication

- Practise – go out of your way to communicate with patients, especially when the subject matter is difficult.
- Try to find somewhere private to talk.
- Identify an appropriate time to engage in talk and ensure that the patient knows how long you might have.
- Get yourself a chair and sit at eye level with the patient; this demonstrates that you have time and brings you down to their physical level.
- Speak clearly, avoiding medical jargon and the use of metaphors.
- If you are giving information, concentrate only on key messages.
- Repeat the key messages.
- Ask the patient to recap to you their understanding of the information.
- Supplement information giving with leaflets, pictures and models; if these are not available, write your own notes for the patient.
- Paraphrase to check what you hear the patient saying: 'Are you saying that … ?'
- Encourage questions; do not say 'Have you any questions?'; instead try 'What questions have you got?'

While developing these communication skills it is useful to reflect on how an interaction went – either alone (perhaps using a reflective diary) or with other people. Of course, the important element of this reflection process is learning from what went well and what did not go so well in order to plan your approach to communicating in the future.

It may seem odd that we concentrate on good communication in a book about evidence-based practice, but there are many benefits that accrue from good communication for both evidence-based nursing and the nurse–patient relationship. Some of these benefits are identified in Table 6.2.

From the point of view of the evidence base of nursing, communication is an absolute necessity. It is the patient who knows not only how they feel physically but also how they feel about their experience of care. Without interacting with the patient we cannot know if what we do as nurses is effective, nor can we know if what we do is appreciated and if the experience of care is good.

Table 6.2: Some of the benefits of good communication

- Better understanding of the condition and treatment options can lead to patients being more able to follow the advice given to them about their care.
- An understanding of what is going on can mean the patient experiences less pain and fewer other symptoms (Hayward, 1979).
- Satisfaction with care can be increased (Maguire and Pitceathly, 2002).
- Patients are more likely to disclose symptoms, which can lead to improved ability to diagnose conditions (Centre for Change and Innovation, 2003).
- Good communication demonstrates that the nurse is patient-centred.
- Subjective data can be collected and used to inform the planning of the patient's care.

Working with other professionals

One of the influences on practice we identified in our model of evidence-based nursing in Chapter 1 was 'views of other professionals'. As we saw in Chapter 5, an understanding and interpretation of the subjective views of others can add greatly to both the amount of knowledge we have and also its depth. Working with other professionals is often termed collaborative practice or interprofessional working and implies something more than the traditional notion of multi-disciplinary working which may be regarded as less integrated.

At its simplest, collaboration is about working together, which implies a commonality of purpose but not a unification of being; it comprises conscious interactions between individuals in order to achieve shared goals, by the overlapping of activities rather than merely working alongside colleagues (Meads et al., 2005). Similarly, interprofessional working has been defined as *how two or more people from the different professions or agencies communicate and cooperate to achieve a common goal* (Øvretveit et al., 1997). As such, interprofessional working is seen as being much broader in its scope than multidisciplinary teamwork and is not just about how practitioners work together but rather about how they manage and plan tasks for the benefit of patients, groups or services.

Within the context of this book, therefore, interprofessional working and collaboration are more about who the individual is rather than what they do – it is one of the dispositions identified in Chapter 1 as being 'other regarding', which supports the notion of allowing the views of other professionals to influence nursing practice. What is important here for the student nurse is that you develop a way of being and of practising nursing which is permanently tuned into the benefits of interprofessional working and the benefits this brings to the patient; it really is not just enough to know about interprofessionality, it is necessary to feel it and allow it to become one of our character traits, our dispositions.

So what are the benefits of interprofessional practice and collaboration for the evidence-based nurse? In the scheme that was presented in Chapter 1, evidence-based nursing is seen as the ability to think judiciously about different strands of information that may collectively be drawn together to create evidence. We saw in Chapter 5 that some of the influences on practice include subjective information and the ability to assimilate this into our understanding of the delivery of care through reflection and reflexivity.

Put simply, the point is this: if we are happy to allow our own experience and reflections to guide the care that we give, then it is perhaps egocentric not to afford this same level of respect to the experiences and reflections of others. There are two good reasons for respecting the experiences and reflections of others: first, we ourselves cannot have experience of everything; second, some individuals have trained in specialist and different areas of care than we, as nurses, have, and this may mean that their understandings of and reflections on care may be more sophisticated and better informed than ours.

This notion of being aware of and open to the knowledge that exists within other professions reflects the nature of nursing, which is essentially an eclectic and holistic application of knowledge that we have gained, and honed, from other disciplines. Put simply, by choosing to listen to and work cooperatively with other professionals, we grow as practitioners and the care we can give patients improves.

There is, of course, a caveat to this acceptance of what others tell us: it must make sense. Like all information accepted as knowledge used to inform the individual evidence base, it is important that we subject it to some scrutiny for ourselves. This is the critical thinking that is alluded to in Chapter 1 and that is discussed again in Chapter 8. This idea of checking also reflects one of the messages in Chapter 5 and earlier in this chapter – that we can use subjective knowledge to validate other subjective knowledge (perhaps other people's views on something we also have a view on) or even to validate more objective forms of knowledge such as the findings of research.

Activity 6.5   *Communication*

Next time you have the opportunity to work with a professional from a different background in the delivery of care, ask them this simple question: 'What are your priorities for the care of this individual and why are these important to you?' Then take some time to reflect on what this means for you as a nurse and how what they said contributes to what it is that you are trying to achieve for the patient – or not.

An outline answer is provided at the end of the chapter.

In essence, then, failing to account for the experience and knowledge of our professional colleagues shuts the door to a very important avenue of learning, which in turn impacts on our ability to develop a holistic evidence base both individually for the patient in front of us now and more generally in the creation of our own bank of professional knowledge.

As well as the concept of learning from professionals from other backgrounds, as nurses we need to continue to learn from each other. The same arguments about why this is important and the need to be critical in our adoption of new knowledge apply here as in the examples of adopting evidence from other professionals.

Barriers to working with other professionals

There are a number of issues that act as barriers to interprofessional collaboration and therefore by default to the development of our own holistic evidence base. These barriers – some of which relate to how we see ourselves as individuals and as nurses and some of which arise as a result of the way in which care is organised – need to be understood before they can be overcome.

We said in Figure 1.1 on p21 that being 'engaged with self' is an important attribute of the evidence-based nurse. But what does this mean?

Being engaged with self is not only about understanding who we are and where we have come from both personally and professionally but also about understanding our motivations, understandings, biases and prejudices. This is not merely about cultural, racial, gender or disability stereotyping; it is about our disposition towards others. Are we willing to engage with others, learn from others, adapt not only our knowledge but perhaps even our values as a result of these interactions? Or are we unable to see the points of view or the understandings that others have and use these to inform not only what we know but perhaps even who we are?

The NMC standards for proficiency require that we *must work in partnership with service users, carers, families, groups, communities and organisations; work with other health and social care professionals collaboratively* (NMC, 2010, p13) and also that we *must use a range of communication skills and technologies to support person-centred care … [and] ensure people receive all the information they need in a language and manner that allows them to make informed choices and share decision-making.* (NMC, 2010, p15).

The point quite simply is this: we cannot show integrity in our practice and in our communication with others unless we actually believe and adopt this value of interprofessional and collaborative practice for real. Integrity requires that this is not a charade, as integrity means acting and communicating in ways that we actually believe!

This does not mean that we should blindly accept what other people tell us or that we should allow patients to make what are essentially bad decisions about their care. The evidence-based morally active nurse takes account of many issues in generating a plan of care using both objective and subjective information.

As well as potential philosophical differences in our approaches to care, other barriers can stand in the way of good collaborative interprofessional care, as shown in Table 6.3. The existence of barriers to interprofessional working have given rise to a number of tragedies over the years, including the deaths of Victoria Climbié and Baby P (Care Quality Commission, 2009). (The Report of the Inquiry into the death of Victoria Climbié can be found on the Department of Health website – **www.dh.gov.uk** – if you put Victoria Climbié into the search box.) Clearly, there are negative consequences of not working in interprofessional ways that extend beyond not creating and operating within a holistic evidence base.

Table 6.3: Some barriers to interprofessional working

- Professional rivalries
- Poor understanding of each other's terminology
- Lack of trust
- Professional labelling and stereotyping
- Traditional hierarchies of care
- Unrealistic expectations
- Lack of resources and management support

Based on the work of Barber et al. (2009).

Strategies for working with other professionals

How, then, can we get to a point at which we work in a more integrated manner with other professionals? What benefits accrue for evidence-based nursing practice if we do? The first of these questions is hard to answer because alone we are unlikely to change ways of working, although we can certainly be role models of collaborative practice. Perhaps by answering the second question – what benefits accrue and for whom? – will enable us to return to the first question and answer it in a meaningful way.

The benefits of collaborative working – certainly within the scheme of evidence-based practice that we are exploring in this book – arise out of the improved ability to deliver person-centred holistic care. Consider Activity 6.6.

Activity 6.6   *Critical thinking*

Gregg is a 59-year-old man who has been admitted to the renal ward needing immediate dialysis. Gregg has type 2 diabetes, which has caused his chronic kidney disease. The diabetes is also responsible for Gregg having poor vision and a diabetic foot ulcer.

List all the specialist staff to whom it might be appropriate to refer Gregg, and state why.

An outline answer is provided at the end of the chapter.

What is clear from the answer to Activity 6.6 is that Gregg will benefit from the input of many different professional groups from within the hospital and potentially from those outside the hospital on discharge. The benefit that interprofessional working brings to Gregg's scenario, assuming the ward nurse co-ordinates his care, is that Gregg receives appropriate and informed care and advice from the person most able to provide it. His care is the best it can be, and all the professionals involved contribute to this. At the centre of this care is Gregg, who is supported by his named nurse. This nurse co-ordinates not only who sees Gregg but also, more importantly, the delivery of the care that is advised, not for him so much as in collaboration with him. Everyone benefits, there is reduced duplication of effort and Gregg gets the care he needs.

How can we as nurses achieve this? Certainly in Activity 6.6 none of this would be possible if the nurse involved was not alert to the possibilities that interprofessional working affords. By role modelling good interprofessional practice the nurse is able to receive information from each of the care professionals involved and use this to plan Gregg's care with him. This receptiveness to the input of other professionals is not received blindly; questions are asked, and the ideas and input received are tested against the nurse's existing understanding and knowledge.

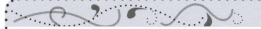

Chapter summary

This chapter has expanded on the nature and purpose of working collaboratively with others to achieve good-quality, evidential care. We have seen that there are a number of barriers to working with others, some of which are created by us and some of which are the result of human nature. We have further identified some important strategies for overcoming these barriers and some good ethical reasons why we must.

Consultation with service users has been framed as a means of improving not only what we do but also the way that we do it and the ways in which care is experienced. We have explored to some extent the need for interprofessional working to achieve high-quality patient care given that the care needs of individuals are increasingly complex. We have seen that evidence-based practice requires a patient-focused (person-centred) approach to care and must be ethical, responding to and overcoming the potential difficulties this poses.

In this chapter there are clearly a number of very big challenges that the busy nurse must face and overcome if they are to achieve care that is responsive to the requirements of the government, the NMC, the research evidence and, most importantly, the patients who we are here to serve.

Activities: Brief outline answers

Activity 6.2: Reflection (page 99)

Being mindful of the opinions, experiences and beliefs of others is a fundamental aspect of moral and ethical behaviour when applied to the process of drawing on evidence to inform nursing practice. Throughout the book we have seen that the evidence base for nursing is not merely about what we do but also about how we go about our work – how it is experienced by others. Within the model of evidence-based nursing there is a need to acknowledge that not everything we do has a basis in scientific or research-based knowledge and that some of the sources of knowledge we use draw upon the experiences and understandings of others. To achieve these lofty goals the nurse therefore needs to be mindful of others while creating for themselves an evidence base in which their practice can be safely and ethically grounded.

Activity 6.5: Communication (page 105)

Nursing goals are often quite broad and represent an attempt to attend to the holistic care of an individual patient. Within these holistic goals will invariably sit a number of single and discrete goals that are shared by other care professionals. For example, the occupational therapist may aim to restore the ability to self-care while the physiotherapist may regard their chief aim as enabling the patient to mobilise safely. Both of these examples reflect the overall aims of nursing, which often relate to enabling the patient to achieve self-care safely. On a broader view, all three approaches are about contributing to care. If we look at the subjective validity of these three views on care we can see that there is a fair degree of overlap, which helps to validate the three different, but converging viewpoints.

Activity 6.6: Critical thinking (page 107)

Gregg might benefit from seeing the following specialist staff.

- The specialist nurses and doctors of the diabetes team would help him get better control of his diabetes.
- The wound care nurse might provide valuable insights into managing Gregg's ulcer.
- The ophthalmologist would prove useful in managing Gregg's deteriorating vision.
- The nephrology consultant would be able to make informed decisions with Gregg about his dialysis and medication relating to his kidney disease.
- The dietician might help Gregg with both his renal and diabetic diet.
- The pharmacist would be useful in helping to rationalise Gregg's medication.
- The renal nurses would be able to discuss dialysis options with Gregg and help him adjust to life on dialysis.
- The renal counsellor might be able to support Gregg in adjusting to his deteriorating health status.
- The social worker could help Gregg apply for appropriate welfare benefits.
- The occupational therapist could help Gregg adapt his home to accommodate his deteriorating vision.

Further reading

Ellis, P (2016) *Understanding research for nursing students* (3rd edn). London: Sage.

See Chapter 6 to gain a better understanding of triangulating data.

Goodman, B and Clemow, R (2010) *Nursing and collaborative practice* (2nd edn). Exeter: Learning Matters.

Contains a great deal of material and activities pertinent to working with others.

Koubel, G and Bungay, H (eds) (2009) *The challenge of person-centred care: an interprofessional perspective.* Basingstoke: Palgrave.

A comprehensive look at the patient as the centre of the care process.

Koubel, G and Bungay, H (eds) (2012) *Rights, risks and responsibilities: interprofessional perspectives.* Basingstoke: Palgrave.

See Chapter 1 for some ideas about what best interests might mean and Chapter 10 about responsibilities when working interprofessionally.

Useful websites

www.caipe.org.uk Website of the Centre for the Advancement of Interprofessional Education.

www.who.int/hrh/resources/framework_action/en Link to the framework for action on interprofessional education and collaborative practice from the World Health Organization.

Chapter 7
Clinical decision-making in evidence-based nursing

Mooi Standing

NMC Standards for Pre-registration Nursing Education

This chapter will address the following competencies:

Domain 3: Nursing practice and decision-making

1. All nurses must use up-to-date knowledge and evidence to assess, plan, deliver and evaluate care, communicate findings, influence change and promote health and best practice. They must make person-centred, evidence-based judgements and decisions, in partnership with others involved in the care process, to ensure high-quality care. They must be able to recognise when the complexity of clinical decisions requires specialist knowledge and expertise, and consult or refer accordingly.

7. All nurses must be able to recognise and interpret signs of normal and deteriorating mental and physical health and respond promptly to maintain or improve the health and comfort of the service user, acting to keep them and others safe.

8. All nurses must provide educational support, facilitation skills and therapeutic nursing interventions to optimise health and well-being. They must promote self-care and management whenever possible, helping people to make choices about their healthcare needs, involving families and carers where appropriate, to maximise their ability to care for themselves.

10. All nurses must evaluate their care to improve clinical decision-making, quality and outcomes, using a range of methods, amending the plan of care, where necessary, and communicating changes to others.

Domain 4: Leadership, management and team working

4. All nurses must be self-aware and recognise how their own values, principles and assumptions may affect their practice. They must maintain their own personal and professional development, learning from experience, through supervision, feedback, reflection and evaluation.

6. All nurses must work independently as well as in teams. They must be able to take the lead in coordinating, delegating and supervising care safely, managing risk and remaining accountable for the care given.

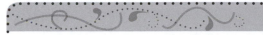

NMC Essential Skills Clusters

This chapter will address the following ESCs:

Cluster: Care, compassion and communication

1. As partners in the care process, people can trust a newly registered graduate nurse to provide collaborative care based on the highest standards, knowledge and competence.

2. People can trust the newly registered graduate nurse to engage in person-centred care empowering people to make choices about how their needs are met when they are unable to meet them for themselves.

8. People can trust the newly registered graduate nurse to gain their consent based on sound understanding and informed choice prior to any intervention and that their rights in decision-making and consent will be respected and upheld.

Cluster: Organisational aspects of care

10. People can trust the newly registered graduate nurse to deliver nursing interventions and evaluate their effectiveness against the agreed assessment and care plan.

12. People can trust the newly registered graduate nurse to respond to their feedback and a wide range of other sources to learn, develop and improve services.

18. People can trust a newly registered graduate nurse to enhance the safety of service users and identify and actively manage risk and uncertainty in relation to people, the environment, self and others.

Chapter aims

After reading this chapter, you will be able to:

*   define clinical decision-making in evidence-based nursing;
*   identify a range of clinical decision-making skills used by nurses;
*   relate decision-making skills to different types of evidence;
*   apply evidence in planned and unplanned nursing decisions;
*   evaluate nursing decisions using the 'PERSON' evaluation tool;
*   understand professional accountability for nursing decisions.

Introduction

This chapter brings together themes from previous chapters about different types of evidence that inform nursing practice to show how they are applied in everyday decisions and actions. Nurses use clinical decision-making skills all the time but they may not always be aware of doing so. From judging how to approach a patient who appears upset about something to taking urgent action to resuscitate a patient who has stopped breathing, effective nursing decisions are life-enhancing and can often be life-saving. Improving nurses' awareness, understanding and expertise in applying clinical decision-making skills is essential in order to provide high-quality, evidence-based nursing. This is reflected in the above Nursing and Midwifery Council's standards for pre-registration nursing education (NMC, 2010), and in a Europe-wide 'Tuning' educational research project that defined a nurse as follows:

> *The nurse is a safe, caring and competent decision maker willing to accept personal and professional accountability for his/her actions and continuous learning. The nurse practises within a statutory framework and code of ethics delivering nursing practice (care) that is appropriately based on research, evidence and critical thinking that effectively responds to the needs of individual clients (patients) and diverse populations.*

> (González and Wagenaar, 2003)

The emphasis placed on nurses as competent decision-makers reflects a shift in expectations of nurses from being mainly practically skilled to being both cognitively and practically skilled, patient-centred professional carers. This involves being answerable and accountable, and being able to explain, justify and defend as necessary the reasons, the supporting evidence and the appropriateness of nursing care decisions and actions. Competent decision-making is an attribute associated with graduate nurses. It also highlights the need for lifelong learning in order for nurses to continually update their knowledge and skills.

This chapter will describe and explore what clinical decision-making in evidence-based nursing means, with reference to relevant theory, research and practical examples. In doing so it will relate clinical decision-making to the different components of the model presented in Figure 1.1 (p21): 'The influences on and dispositions of an evidence-based nurse'. A 'PERSON' evaluation tool (Standing, 2014) will also be presented with which to evaluate nurses' evidence-based clinical decision-making in caring for patients.

Clinical decision-making skills and associated processes

Clinical decision-making is commonly associated with diagnosing illness and prescribing treatment. However, it is more than that, because unless you switch your brain off when you go to work in a clinical area, everything you do involves making a decision, for example, how you manage your time, interact with patients, relate to other healthcare team members and carry out clinical procedures. To research nurses' decision-making processes, a group of 20 new nursing students were asked to keep reflective journals about their experience and understanding of acquiring and applying clinical decision-making skills for four years, including their first year as registered nurses. In a series of four interviews, ten perceptions of clinical decision-making skills in nursing were identified (see Table 7.1).

Table 7.1: Perceptions of clinical decision-making skills from student nurse to staff nurse

Collaborative	Sharing, consulting and agreeing decisions with others, i.e. patients, relatives, nursing colleagues, mentors, managers, supervisors, other health professionals, and other agencies if appropriate, e.g. social worker, home warden, charity worker.
Experience and intuition	Recognising similarities between present and past situations and being guided in what to do by what seems to have been effective before (and avoiding any previous mistakes), e.g. learning how to attend, listen to, communicate and empathise with others in a relaxed but purposeful way that focuses on their needs.
Confidence	Developing self-assurance from previous achievements, knowledge and skills, plus the strength of supporting evidence that enables explanation, justification and defence of decisions and actions.
Systematic	Using a purposeful, methodical, disciplined problem-solving cycle, including identifying and assessing problems, setting goals and making plans, implementing and evaluating (revising as needed) interventions.
Prioritising	Assessing and managing risks: dealing with urgent before non-urgent patient needs; avoiding causing any further harm to patients.
Observation	Making constant use of senses to look, listen or feel if patients need assistance; monitoring vital signs; recording response to treatment; reviewing results of investigations; reporting any concerns promptly.
Standardised	Applying NHS Trust policies/procedures, evidence-based clinical guidelines and assessment tools, and agreed care plans.
Reflective	Undertaking ongoing individual/collective review of experience to identify insights and address knowledge gaps to inform future care.
Ethical sensitivity	Checking patients are informed and consent to care; communicating 'bad news' sensitively; and maintaining duty of care in ethical dilemmas.
Accountability	Ensuring actions are defensible, are in patients' best interests and comply with NMC Code, local policy, relevant legislation.

Source: Standing, 2005.

Table 7.1 implies that clinical decision-making in nursing is very complex. This is because it involves continually combining and applying many different processes in anticipating and responding to the needs of those in your care through timely, well-informed, justifiable actions throughout a period of duty. In the following case study, a student nurse coming to the end of her second Adult Branch placement reflects on an incident in which she felt she had to take the initiative to support the wife of a patient.

> ### Case study: The patient's wife
>
> *A gentleman was scheduled for an operation to remove cancer from his bowel and create a colostomy (permanent opening in his abdomen) where a special bag would be attached to collect and dispose of faeces for the rest of his life. He was, naturally, anxious about having such major surgery and his wife came in to comfort him before he went to theatre.*
>
> *When it was time for him to go, I said to his wife, 'You can go down with him if you like. I'll show you where it is.' I took her along and checked that the receiving theatre staff were happy for her to stay until the anaesthetic was given. When she returned to the ward she sat in a chair by the empty space where her husband's bed had been, looking very worried. I said, 'Are you OK?' She burst into tears, and I knew she needed someone to spend time with her, so I said, 'Look, I'll go and make a cup of tea.' I pulled the curtains round and we had a cup of tea together (I don't know whether I should have had one but it felt more natural having a cup of tea together) and a chat. She told me about him and about herself and her family, and after a few tears I put my arm around her. She really was grateful afterwards and said, 'You know, I really needed someone to talk to.' I look back on that and I am so glad I sat and spoke to that woman and that I knew she needed someone to talk to. It could be my mother, you see, and I would hate to think that nobody sat and comforted her. It was basic human rights, common-sense stuff. A year ago I might not have done that, but I have grown in confidence.*

Applying the ten perceptions of clinical decision-making skills to the case study

It is important that nurses can question, examine, explain, justify and defend their decisions and actions when required. The ten perceptions of clinical decision-making skills identified in Table 7.1 offer a useful framework to analyse the nursing student's clinical decision-making skills in the case study, as follows:

Observation: The student nurse noticed how anxious the patient looked prior to surgery, how worried the wife looked on returning to the ward, and how she seemed to benefit from talking to someone.

Experience and intuition: The student nurse knew it was possible for relatives to accompany patients to theatre when she suggested it, and she sensed this was appropriate as the patient was anxious and seemed comforted by the wife's presence. She also understood that the wife had to suppress her own fears about the outcome of surgery and had nobody else to confide in about this.

Collaborative: The student nurse worked in partnership with the patient and his wife to reduce his level of stress prior to surgery. She ensured that the receiving theatre team agreed for the wife to stay until the anaesthetic was given, and she made herself available to support the wife if needed.

Ethical sensitivity: The student nurse extended a duty of care to include the wife as well as the patient in recognising her fears about the seriousness and long-term implications of his condition. She was aware it was not accepted practice to stop for a cup of tea and a chat with a relative on a busy ward, but she judged it was appropriate as it was an effective way to offer support.

Prioritising: The student nurse knew the patient's needs were being addressed in theatre, she had no one else to prepare for surgery, and she recognised the wife might need an opportunity to talk.

Standardised: Preoperative procedures (consent, bath, fasting, medication to relax, check identity tag, vital signs, remove dentures) would have been followed, ensuring the gentleman was ready for surgery.

Systematic: The student nurse demonstrated skilful use of informative, supportive and cathartic interventions (Heron, 2001): in letting the wife know she could accompany her husband to theatre (**informative interventions**); in acknowledging her anxieties, concerns and need to talk (**supportive**); and in giving her permission to express her feelings by asking directly 'Are you OK?' and then reassuring her that she had time to listen (**cathartic**).

Accountability: The supervising staff nurse is technically accountable for care given by the student, but their main priority was pre- and post-operative patient care. The student's sense of responsibility for supporting the patient's wife is endorsed by the NMC Code, which states that you should *recognise when people are anxious or in distress and respond compassionately and politely* (NMC, 2015, p5).

Reflective: The student nurse applied **reflection-in-action** in taking the initiative to facilitate the wife accompanying the patient to theatre and in responding to her apparent distress when she returned. Looking back, she used **reflection-on-action** in affirming the importance of supporting relatives.

Confidence: The student nurse had grown in confidence in her decision-making and interpersonal skills in recognising and addressing the wife's unmet needs, and achieving a successful outcome.

Having applied the ten perceptions of clinical decision-making to review the nursing student's interventions in the case study, it begs the question – so what? Is it a case of over-theorising and over-analysing a relatively straightforward and common-sense example of good nursing practice? Or does the application of such frameworks (informed by and developed from research evidence) tell us something important about the nature of clinical decision-making in evidence-based nursing practice?

Activity 7.1	*Critical thinking*

One way for you to assess the usefulness of the ten perceptions of clinical decision-making is to consider whether or not they promote the development and application of the essential 'dispositions of the evidence-based nurse' identified in Chapter 1 (Figure 1.1). These are listed below. Look again at the ten perceptions of clinical decision-making and try to match them to any of the dispositions you think they relate to, with reference to appropriate examples from the case study where possible.

continued …

Dispositions of the evidence-based nurse	Perceptions of clinical decision-making relating to the dispositions	Examples in case study of linking the dispositions and perceptions
• Other regarding • Engaged with self • Questioning • Reflective • Reflexive • Creative thinker • Critical thinker • Morally active		

Some possible outline answers are provided at the end of the chapter.

So far this chapter has described different aspects (perceptions) of clinical decision-making and suggested that they relate to different qualities (dispositions) of nurses in evidence-based practice. Later on in the chapter the ten perceptions of clinical decision-making will be related to the different types of evidence identified in Chapter 1. Before moving on to that, it is worth spending a bit more time thinking about other characteristics of clinical decision-making highlighted in the case study. The case study illustrates a contrast between nursing decisions and actions that are planned and those that are unplanned. Preoperative nursing care of the patient would have been a well-planned and standardised procedure, whereas noticing and responding to the patient's and his wife's fear and anxiety was a spontaneous or unplanned reaction applying experience and intuition. The relatively high level of contact nurses have with patients, relatives, friends and carers (compared to many other professions) means that they get more opportunities for both planned and unplanned clinical decision-making. Are you aware of how much time you spend on planned as opposed to unplanned nursing care?

Activity 7.2   *Reflection*

Identify a day in your clinical placement to do a 'time and motion' study of everything you do from the moment you arrive to the moment you leave the clinical area. Take a notebook with you to record events and their duration during your shift if possible (so you don't have to try to recall everything at the end of the day). Review the day's activities and calculate how much time was spent on planned (e.g. agreed care plan) versus unplanned (e.g. responding to situations that arise) decisions and associated patient care. Match each example to the ten perceptions of clinical decision-making skills as appropriate for both planned and unplanned care. Reflect on whether the ten perceptions apply equally to planned and unplanned decisions and related nursing care.

Some possible answers can be found at the end of the chapter.

Sometimes nursing interventions need to combine elements of both planned and unplanned decision-making. For example, our duty to ensure patient safety means that potential unexpected events such as a fire, an accident in a clinical area, a medical emergency, or dealing with an aggressive incident must be anticipated. Contingency plans such as a fire drill must be made, ready to put into effect when required. It is important that you discuss with your clinical mentor what is expected of you and your role in such circumstances. Ask to see policies and procedures for managing such events so you are familiar with them and take part in any drills and training events to practise procedures and help to develop the necessary skills.

Activity 7.3   *Research and finding out*

Look through the various emergency guidelines and procedures in your clinical placement and see if you can identify examples of the ten perceptions of clinical decision-making skills being applied.

Identify any of the ten perceptions of clinical decision-making skills that you feel should be applied in all situations (including carefully planned care, spontaneous unplanned care and implementing procedures for emergencies) and write down why you think they are important. Check whether your fellow students, clinical colleagues and mentor agree or disagree with your choices.

Some possible answers can be found at the end of the chapter.

Defining clinical decision-making in nursing

Decision-making involves choosing what action to take from the available alternatives and then carrying it out. In its most basic form it means choosing to do something or choosing not to do it, for example, washing hands before cooking a meal or not (in which case not washing hands is an alternative action, albeit passive) and saying 'yes' or 'no' when someone offers you a cup of tea. Decision-making, therefore, employs thinking skills to exercise judgement in assessing the benefits of possible options and choosing a preferred option that is then acted upon. Clinical decision-making refers to decisions made by health professionals in the course of their work in promoting health, diagnosing or treating disease, relieving suffering, and caring for patients. Becoming skilled in clinical decision-making requires the application of a range of evidence regarding: patient concerns, physical and human resources within healthcare contexts, understanding health and illness, developing expertise in applying therapeutic approaches, a commitment to enhance the well-being of those in your care, and fulfilling the requirements of the relevant professional body.

Clinical decision-making in nursing refers to any decisions made by nurses in choosing how to deliver care to patients for whom they are responsible. The Nursing and Midwifery Council is the professional body that specifies education requirements for entry to the register as a qualified nurse and for maintaining registration status. It also regulates the profession through publishing a code of conduct that nurses must comply with or face potential disciplinary action. For example: *We can take action if registered nurses or midwives fail to uphold the Code. In serious cases, this can include removing them from the register* (NMC, 2015, p2). Making the wrong clinical decisions is, therefore, not only potentially harmful to patients, it may also call into question your continuing practice as a nurse. Learning about, developing and applying effective clinical decision-making skills is vital for the well-being of patients, and nurses' capacity to demonstrate that decisions are justified. The following definition summarises key elements of clinical decision-making in nursing.

> *Clinical decision-making is a complex process involving observation, information processing, critical thinking, evaluating evidence, applying relevant knowledge, problem solving skills, reflection and clinical judgement to select the best course of action which optimises a patient's health and minimises any potential harm. The role of the clinical decision-maker in nursing is, therefore, to be professionally accountable for accurately assessing patients' needs using appropriate sources of information, and planning nursing interventions that address problems and which they are competent to perform.*
>
> (Standing, 2005, 2007, 2010)

This definition emphasises that clinical decisions:

- are patient-centred in anticipating and responding to patients'/service users' needs to address their health problems;

- involve identifying, reviewing and applying relevant information from different sources, for example, observations, the patient's story, clinical guidelines, theory and research evidence;

- require the application of cognitive skills such as problem solving, critical thinking, reflection and judgement in selecting the best option;

- are associated with delivering competent, effective nursing care for which nurses are accountable.

In this way clinical decision-making reflects the notion of evidence-based nursing, as described and advocated throughout this book. These skills are central to nurses' professional identity, as stated in the definition of a nurse (González and Wagenaar, 2003) presented at the beginning of this chapter. In Activity 7.4 you are asked to apply aspects of the above definition to reflect on your own experience of clinical decision-making.

Activity 7.4   *Reflection*

Next time you are in a clinical practice setting, make a point of noting down all the decisions that relate to patient care that *you* have to make during your shift. Later, when you have time, reflect on these decisions, then try to answer the following questions.

1. In what way were your decisions relevant to the needs of the patients you cared for?
2. What type of evidence did you refer to and how did this influence your decision-making?

---

continued ...

3.   What types of thinking skills did you apply?

4.   How did you evaluate the outcomes of your decisions?

As this is based on your own reflections, there is no outline answer at the end of the chapter.

Applying different types of evidence in nursing decisions

Evidence refers to information that is used to support particular beliefs, decisions and actions. It can be sensory: for example, feeling tired and hungry at the end of 'a long day' at work and deciding to stop at a favourite eating place on the way home rather than cook something yourself. It can be emotional: for example, feeling sad or angry about something that happened and deciding to talk to a sympathetic friend to 'get it off your chest'. It can be practical: for example, you notice that your front door has begun to squeak annoyingly when opened or closed so you decide to oil its hinges. It can be theoretical: for example, planning a holiday abroad and deciding to read up on the history, customs and culture, and places of interest to visit. It can be technological: for example, needing to ensure information on the home computer is not lost if the system 'crashes' and deciding to install a back-up external hard drive. It can also be scientific, for example, understanding that water conducts electricity and deciding to dry your hands and body before switching on the hairdryer to reduce the risk of an electric shock. In the above examples personal decisions, subsequent actions and their potential consequences are prompted by knowledge and understanding derived from a wide range of information sources or types of evidence. The same is true of nursing decisions.

Earlier chapters looked in detail at different types of evidence in nursing. Chapter 1 summarised these in Figure 1.1, 'The influences on and dispositions of an evidence-based nurse' (p21). In order to see how different types of evidence may influence nursing decisions, Table 7.2 suggests possible matches with the ten perceptions of clinical decision-making skills described earlier.

Table 7.2: Different types of evidence informing clinical decision-making skills in nursing	
Evidence influencing practice	**Associated clinical decision-making skills**
Research evidence	Systematic, standardised
Practice knowledge	Observation, reflective
Experience	Experience and intuition, confidence
Policy	Prioritising, standardised
Resources	Prioritising, accountability
Patient preference	Collaborative, ethical sensitivity
Views of other professionals	Collaborative, experience and intuition
Ethics	Ethical sensitivity, accountability
Law	Accountability, standardised

Applying research evidence to systematic and standardised decision-making

Research evidence is often seen as the essential basis of high-quality, evidence-based healthcare because it involves rigorous testing of the validity and reliability of methods used and reported findings, which are open to critical scrutiny and testing by others (see Chapters 3 and 4). This scientific (physical and social) approach to generating new knowledge has influenced the development of systematic problem solving and associated decision-making – for example, the nursing process (ongoing cycle of assessment, planning, implementation and evaluation of care). In many clinical areas the use of the nursing process is standardised, meaning it is adopted as a framework for all nurses to use in delivering and recording care. To guide nurses in targeting systematic care, the nursing process is often used in conjunction with the Activities of Living model (Roper et al., 2000; Holland et al., 2008) to assess patients' abilities and needs in 12 areas (maintaining a safe environment, communicating, breathing, eating and drinking, eliminating, personal cleansing and dressing, controlling body temperature, mobilising, working and playing, expressing sexuality, sleeping and preparing for dying). In effect, this is a checklist of patients' general physical, psychological and social health and well-being to help nurses provide comprehensive person-centred care in partnership with patients.

Research evidence also informs clinical guidelines produced by the National Institute of Health and Care Excellence (NICE) in caring for particular patients with specific needs and health problems. It is highly likely that there is a relevant NICE clinical guideline relating to whichever area of practice you are working. NICE clinical guidelines are being continually developed, applied to patient care and updated.

Case study: Care of patients who have learning disabilities and suffer from epilepsy

The Clinical Guideline 'CG137 – Epilepsies: diagnosis and management' (NICE, 2012) assists nurses and other health professionals in caring for adults and children suffering from various forms of epilepsy (neurological abnormality associated with involuntary seizures (fits) and/or loss of consciousness). People with learning disabilities are on average 20 times more likely to suffer from epilepsy than the general population. A study was therefore set up to compare care, for this group of vulnerable patients, before and after the previous edition (CG20) of these guidelines were implemented. The results of the study are summarised below.

Implementing NICE guideline CG20 for the management of epilepsy in a learning disability service

	Before implementation	After implementation
Proportion of patients whose seizures were accurately described and classified	6%	83%
Proportion where frequency of seizures was recorded	81%	100%

continued ...

	Before implementation	After implementation
Proportion where severity of seizures was recorded	57%	100%
Proportion of changes made to seizure diagnosis	0%	76%
Proportion of individualised risk assessment carried out	4.5%	100%
Medical consultations led to changes in treatment plans	50%	91%

Source: NICE (2007).

The above case study illustrates how evidence-based, standardised clinical guidelines can help healthcare practitioners to work more systematically in identifying and managing health problems. It indicated that assessment of patients' symptoms became much more accurate and comprehensive, which in turn informed changes to patients' diagnosis, risk management and medical treatment. Such guidelines not only inform medical treatment, they also influence nurses' decision-making and offer information for service users and/or their families to understand the options available to them. It also shows that clinical guidelines are always evolving following a review of their application in order to provide up-to-date evidence-based care.

Activity 7.5   *Decision-making*

Although epilepsy may be more common in people with learning disabilities, it can affect anyone, including people with mental health problems, children and adults throughout the population. Whichever pathway you are practising in, it is therefore important that you know how to assess and manage various health risks associated with this condition. Use the 12 areas (listed above) in the Activities of Living model (Roper et al., 2000; Holland et al., 2008) as a checklist for a risk assessment of someone having a 'grand mal' epileptic fit and say how you would manage the risks during and following tonic (involuntary muscle rigidity) and clonic (involuntary alternating muscle contractions) phases of the seizure.

Some possible answers can be found at the end of the chapter.

Applying practice knowledge to observation and reflective decision-making

While research evidence is usually documented, made explicit and widely disseminated, practice knowledge refers to localised, context-specific skills and tacit understanding, for example, the **embedded** customs and practices that distinguish one clinical placement from another. Practice knowledge includes technical skills such as the dexterity to do an aseptic wound dressing, inter-personal skills in being attentive and listening to patients' concerns, and noticing changes in behaviour that signal someone needs attention (as the student did in the patient's wife case study). In the following case study a surgical nurse intervenes when a patient complains of pain in a limb he no longer has.

Case study: Phantom pain

Following surgery, a gentleman who smoked heavily for 40 years, and who suffers from peripheral vascular disease (poor circulation affecting feet and legs) and diabetes, is distressed by pains he feels come from his right foot following below-knee amputation of his right leg, which had been gangre-nous. Through reflection-in-action the surgical nurse understands that this is a 'phantom pain' commonly experienced by amputees as real, sometimes severe pain, which they may find disturbing. The gentleman is offered painkillers as prescribed, and is reassured that what he is experiencing is not unusual, that the pains should gradually subside, and that the science behind this phenomenon is not yet fully understood.

In reflecting back on encounters with patients ('reflection-on-action') nurses can try to relate their clinical experience to relevant theory or research evidence. However, in order to direct a search you need to ask questions, based on observation and practical understanding of patients' needs. In relation to the above example we might ask, 'Might visualisation and virtual massage of amputated limbs help to relieve "phantom pains" experienced by amputees?' Similarly, if appropriate research-based procedures are discovered and implemented, their effectiveness needs to be evaluated, and this also requires the application of practice knowledge using obser-vation and communication skills to reflect on care outcomes with patients. Reflection-on-action may also help to identify valuable practice knowledge, or skills that are usually invisibly embedded in clinical contexts, and then make them explicit.

Activity 7.6   *Reflection*

Identify a clinical placement that you have been allocated to and try to identify specific practice knowledge you associate with experienced nurses in that particular area of patient care.

- What technical and practical knowledge and skills do the nurses apply?
- What interpersonal and communication skills do you notice the nurses using?
- What observation skills do nurses demonstrate in that clinical area?
- What examples of the nurses' reflective clinical decision-making have you witnessed?
- Talk to your mentor about how you can develop your practice knowledge and related skills.

As this is activity is based on your own reflection, there is no outline answer at the end of the chapter.

Applying experience to experience and intuition and confidence in decision-making

Experience refers to an accumulation of personal, **embodied** understanding that incorporates an individual's unique interpretation of their role as a nurse; interpersonal relationships with patients, staff and others; theoretical and research input; and influential life events. Connecting these disparate influences defines a nurse's personal and professional identity, which the individual draws upon in subconsciously recognising patterns in information cues to facilitate their intuitive judgement. In a sense this is what happens between people who have intimate mutual understanding and, without prompting, know what the other person is thinking or feeling. Developing and confidently using this skill as a nurse in quickly assessing a crisis situation, understanding what needs to done and organising an effective, speedy resolution is associated with expert practitioners (Benner, 1984). This is the most difficult type of decision to explain because it may be based on a hunch or feeling that is only justified where there is a positive outcome. However, this type of decision is prone to error; for example, you might believe a parent who says her child tripped while playing, only to discover later it was a non- accidental injury from physical abuse. It is, therefore, advisable to test out intuitions, for example, by seeking out a second opinion from an experienced colleague.

Activity 7.7   *Communication*

Test out your intuitive abilities with a group of colleagues at college or in the clinical area.

- Each person privately thinks of a living creature they feel they can strongly identify with.
- Everyone writes (in BLOCK CAPITALS to reduce handwriting recognition) the name of their chosen creature on the same type/size paper and all the names are put into a hat.
- Someone makes a list of all the creatures identified in the hat for everyone to share (if two people happen to identify the same creature then list it twice).
- Each person then privately writes down which group member they feel most closely characterises each living creature.
- Everyone goes through the list of creatures together to see how many guesses were right and how many were wrong.

As this activity is based on your own engagement with the activity, there is no outline answer at the end of the chapter.

Applying policy to prioritising and standardised decision-making

Following devolution and further decentralisation of UK government responsibilities in 2012, NHS policy and related priorities are decided by the Department of Health in England and by the respective governments of Scotland, Wales and Northern Ireland. For example, Jeremy

Hunt, Secretary of State for Health, identified the following priorities to improve people's health in England:

1. preventing people from dying prematurely by improving mortality rates;

2. improving the standard of care throughout the system;

3. improving treatment and care of people with dementia;

4. bringing the technology revolution to the NHS to help people, especially those with long term conditions, manage their health and care.

(DH, 2014)

Helping people live longer, healthier lives is a recurring theme in health policy. The NHS Plan (DH, 2000) identified that 75 per cent of deaths in those under the age of 75 were caused by cardiovascular disease, cancer, mental illness/suicide and accidents, so it set targets to significantly reduce mortality rates in these areas by 2010. All patients attending accident and emergency centres had to be assessed, treated and discharged/transferred within four hours. The Plan also called for more health promotion, such as nurses giving patients information and advice on dieting, exercising and self-care such as managing pain. Translating health policy into prioritising and standardised decision-making is enabled by National Institute for Health Research (NIHR) projects such as how to improve the quality of life of dementia sufferers and carers. The NIHR therefore produces research which is incorporated within evidence-based NICE clinical guidelines to improve the quality of patient care. However, these scientific and technological developments are of limited use unless they are applied in a way that benefits and values patients as unique individuals to whom healthcare practitioners are accountable. This point is reinforced by health policy which requires nurses to apply the '6Cs' (Care, Compassion, Competence, Communication, Courage, Commitment) when caring for patients and service users (DH, 2012b).

Applying resources to prioritising and accountability in decision-making

A potential problem in setting health targets that encourage more patients to be treated in less time is ensuring there are sufficient human and physical resources to meet the increased demand, and provide high-quality care. After all, the health targets are intended to enhance public health. Sadly, evidence emerged that patient safety and the quality of healthcare received was compromised due to NHS Trusts being preoccupied with the pursuit of prescribed targets. In 2007 the Healthcare Commission (an NHS 'watchdog', replaced in 2009 by the Care Quality Commission) reported 90 deaths from *Clostridium difficile* infection in one NHS Trust during the period 2004–2006. It concluded that the Trust had failed to monitor, report, recognise or respond appropriately to the risks posed by the life-threatening bug as it was not on their list of targets. There was inadequate leadership in infection control, not enough nurses for a high (90 per cent) bed occupancy rate, a lack of isolation rooms to contain the outbreak, a lack of uptake on training programmes, and unacceptable standards of hygiene. Patients who had acute diarrhoea from the infection were allegedly told to evacuate in the bed as no one could attend to them, and then they were left soiled for long periods. The *Clostridium difficile* outbreak came to light because of high mortality rates. The Trust's senior management personnel were held accountable for system failings. Clearly, policy, priorities and resource management by NHS Trusts impact upon nursing decisions and the quality of care provided. However, nurses must also bear some of the shame for the misdirected and fragmented healthcare systems that badly failed patients they were duty bound to protect.

Similar catastrophic healthcare failures were uncovered by a public inquiry into the Mid Staffordshire NHS Foundation Trust (Francis, 2013) following patients' and relatives' complaints of appalling care which were substantiated by high mortality rates. The stark realisation that the NHS itself was 'sick' meant that urgent reform was needed. This has resulted in the Health and Social Care Act 2012 and 2015 which aims to give patients a voice, more choice and better quality care. Clinical Commissioning Groups (guided by an independent NHS Commissioning Board) comprising GPs and others have responsibility for commissioning healthcare services relevant to the needs of the local population. They replaced Strategic Health Authorities and Primary Care Trusts to reduce bureaucracy and associated administration costs and refocus resources on delivering safe and effective, high-quality, person-centred, evidence-based care responsive to the needs of the local community.

Applying patient preference to collaborative and ethical sensitivity in decision-making

In the circumstances described above, patients' preferences were evidently disregarded as there was a failure to provide them with an acceptable standard of care, their complaints were ignored, and the serious implications of unusually high mortality rates were denied. This is in spite of the fact that the Department of Health and NHS Trusts advocate high-quality patient-centred care, greater treatment choice, invite verbal, written or online feedback from patients about their experiences, and have policies in place that are supposed to deal with patients' or relatives' complaints promptly and thoroughly. It is, therefore, important for nurses not simply to listen to patients' preferences or queries regarding their care but to respond appropriately in respecting their views and addressing their concerns.

In some situations patient preference is not catered for because of financial constraints and geographical variations in policy. For example, new drugs prolonging lives of those suffering from cancer are not available in some NHS Trusts because they are considered too expensive, but in others the same drugs are freely available. Sometimes patients do not want the NHS to prolong their lives and refuse treatment, presenting healthcare professionals with an ethical dilemma.

Case study: Refusal of treatment

A frail 98-year-old patient, who has outlived all her relatives and friends, stopped eating a week ago and says she does not want to be fed by any alternative means. If the healthcare team do not intervene, they will be respecting her wishes but contributing to her starvation and potential premature death. If they decide to feed her with supplements via intravenous infusion, they will be going against her wishes but will probably extend her sad and lonely life.

Activity 7.8   *Reflection*

If you were a member of the healthcare team in the case study above, which of the two options would you support and what reasons can you give to justify your choice of action?

The actual answer reached by the team is referred to in the next section for your information.

Sometimes patients take more direct action to end their lives. For example, a young man being treated for depression in an acute mental health unit says goodnight to the new night nurse and goes to bed. When the nurse goes round checking on patients an hour later he discovers the young man dead underneath the covers having tied a plastic bag over his head. The nurse feels terribly guilty for not taking more time to talk to the patient and for not checking on him sooner. These feelings are exacerbated as the police and coroner investigate the death (ruling out homicide), by the parents' grief at losing their son when they thought he was being safely looked after, and in having to describe and explain his actions to hospital managers.

Activity 7.9   *Reflection*

Do you agree with the nurse that he could have prevented the young man's suicide if he had been more vigilant? Do you think the nurse was particularly negligent in the standard of care offered? What evidence might have been helpful in alerting the nurse to observe the young man closely?

There are some possible answers and thoughts at the end of the chapter.

Applying views, experience and intuition to collaborative decision-making

The dilemma presented by the elderly lady refusing food requires careful consideration and collaboration between the patient, nurses, doctors and managers. One nurse had formed a good relationship with the patient through spending time with her, listening and talking to her about her past, how she is feeling now, her likes and dislikes, and her refusal to accept nutrients. Sometimes the lady agreed to sip a cup of tea or, with encouragement, to nibble on a biscuit, but it was not enough to sustain her. In contributing to a team discussion the nurse said she did not agree with intravenous feeding because it would upset the lady and deny her the dignity of choosing how to spend the remainder of her life. Others felt uncomfortable that this could be seen as neglect and that every effort should be made to keep her alive. Some wondered whether the lady might not be mentally competent to make a decision and thought the team ought to make one for her in the absence of relatives. However, the nurse argued that the lady was quite lucid, not confused, sad but not severely depressed, and it would be uncaring to force her into actions that would prolong her life against her wishes. The team finally agreed that they would respect the patient's wishes by not feeding her artificially (intravenously) but that the nurses would continue offering her food and drink, and someone to talk to. Pooling experiences and views to debate patient care in this way is a valuable way of promoting effective teamwork. Teamwork enables learning from different perspectives and disciplines, feeling valued and recognised by interprofessional colleagues, and co-ordinating and integrating an effective system of care delivery tailored to the individual patient's unique needs.

Activity 7.10   *Research and finding out*

Research the Tony Bland case (the case of a young man in a coma from crush injuries from the Hillsborough Football Stadium disaster in 1989), which set a legal precedent classifying artificial nutrition as medical treatment that doctors (in collaboration with others) could decide whether to give or not. The House of Commons Medical Treatment (Prevention of Euthanasia) Bill (2000) is a useful information source.

As this activity involves your own research, there is no outline answer at the end of the chapter.

Applying ethics to ethical sensitivity and accountability in decision-making

As described in Figure 1.1, ethical principles (respect for human rights, commitment to good practice, avoidance of harm and treatment of all patients fairly) underpin high-quality, patient-centred, evidence-based nursing. As referred to earlier, the NMC is the professional body that sets out the ethical code of conduct that nurses in the UK must comply with. Good practice – for example, the student nurse being sensitive to the wife of a cancer patient in the first case study in this chapter – exemplifies the application of ethical principles, while poor practice – for example, patients being left in badly soiled bed-linen – is in breach of all the above principles, and the Code (NMC, 2015). In order to maintain public trust and the right to remain on the nursing register, nurses must always conduct themselves in a caring, professional, well-informed and competent manner. Where this is found not to be the case nurses are held to account for their behaviour and disciplined, which can include being removed from the NMC register and forfeiting the right to work as a registered nurse.

Case studies: Examples of misconduct

These are examples of nurses who received 'Striking Off Orders' from the NMC register at the Conduct and Competence Committee hearings (September 2015) when their fitness to practise was found to be currently impaired.

- *An adult medical unit nurse failed to carry out appropriate safety checks prior to the administration of blood resulting in the wrong blood transfusion being given to a patient. The nurse also failed to undertake and/or document appropriate observations of the patient after administering the wrong blood transfusion.*

continued ...

- *A learning disabilities community nurse failed to visit certain patients in the community when it was her duty to do so. The nurse failed to record visits or write appropriate care plans for patients who had been seen. The nurse also failed to ensure that risk assessment documents were completed and failed to request further diagnostic tests and a CT head scan needed to assess risks to patients' health.*

- *A mental health nurse was convicted under the Sexual Offences Act 2003 and imprisoned for: (i) Causing or inciting a child to engage in sexual activity – contrary to section 10(1); (ii) Meeting a child following sexual grooming – contrary to section 15(1); (iii) Sexual activity with a child – contrary to section 9(1). The nurse met the victim at an amateur dramatic group and the crimes occurred outside of work but the serious nature of the offences meant the nurse was found unsuitable to remain on the register.*

- *A children's nurse prepared a child for surgery including administering premedication despite knowing that the child had recently eaten which made it unsafe to operate at that time. The nurse failed to carry out appropriate postoperative observations. The nurse also failed to escalate concerns to medical staff when a child's Paediatric Advanced Warning Score (PAWS) of 4 indicated that this was necessary.*

Source: www.nmc-uk.org/concerns-nurses-midwives/hearings-and-outcomes/schedule-and-outcomes/september-2015-new/

Applying law to accountability and standardised decision-making

The NMC is empowered under the terms of Nursing and Midwifery Order 2001 legislation to safeguard the health and well-being of the public and regulate the profession. Similarly, nursing students have to demonstrate good health, good character and fitness to practise, and to declare any police cautions, charges or criminal convictions to ensure patients are protected (NMC, 2009).

The law, specifically the Health and Safety at Work Act 1974, can protect all nurses in the workplace by requiring employers to take measures (training, equipment, procedures) to control risks to their health and safety. Employees also have a responsibility to report safety concerns; arguably, the nurses at the NHS Trust referred to earlier had sufficient grounds to report serious health risks regarding infection-control systems, procedures and associated staffing problems.

The law can also be used to protect all patients. For example, the Data Protection Act 1998 (OPSI, 1998) requires confidential patient information to be kept securely and accessed only by authorised personnel. Nurses need to think about the implications of this legislation in their everyday practice, for example, when asking patients about their personal details, given that the rise in identity fraud highlights risks associated with a lack of privacy.

> ### Scenario
>
> *A patient attends an outpatient clinic for an appointment with a consultant to review recent tests of her heart and lung function. The waiting room is full of other patients, but the experienced nurse loudly and unceremoniously asks her to confirm her full name, address, date of birth, telephone number, work contact details and next of kin, then weighs her and announces the result for all to hear.*

In the above scenario the patient's confidential information was not kept securely and was accessible to non-authorised personnel contrary to the Data Protection Act 1998. It was also a breach of section 5.1 of the Code, 'respect a person's right to privacy in all aspects of their care' (NMC, 2015, p6). The experienced nurse should have therefore ensured the interview was conducted discreetly and sensitively.

Under the terms of the Freedom of Information Act, 2000, the public have the right to see any records made by nurses or others regarding their care. Hence, it is important for nurses to remember that relevant sections of case notes and reflective portfolios they have compiled could be accessed and scrutinised by patients and their legal representatives.

Some laws relate to specific groups of service users. For example, the Children Act 1989 (OPSI, 1989) specifies that if you have reason to suspect that a child has been physically, emotionally or sexually abused, you must report it straightaway to social services who are obliged to investigate, and if necessary remove the child to a place of safety. With mentally ill patients there may be a double risk regarding self-harm or sometimes a possibility of harming others. The Mental Health Act 1983 specifies criteria for the voluntary or compulsory treatment of patients according to the perceived type, level and duration of risk to themselves or others, to protect both patients and the public. The Mental Capacity Act 2005 protects people who are unable to make decisions and requires nurses and others who have a duty of care to act in their best interests.

Evaluating evidence-based nursing decisions using 'PERSON'

We have seen that the ten perceptions of clinical decision-making identified by nurses (Standing, 2005) can be related to the nine different forms of evidence described in this book. This may be helpful to you if you are asked to explain the rationale and evidence-base of your own nursing decisions. Registered nurses are obliged to ask themselves this question every time they make a clinical decision because they are professionally accountable for delivering safe and effective person-centred, evidence-based patient care. The **'PERSON' evaluation tool** has been developed to help nurses and midwives evaluate their clinical decisions.

Whichever perceptions of clinical decision-making that you are applying (e.g. 'collaborative', 'ethical sensitivity') you can evaluate your decisions using the 'PERSON' evaluation tool. Similarly, 'PERSON' offers a structure to harness the dispositions of the evidence-based nurse (Chapter 1) to evaluate your clinical decision-making. For example, the 'other regarding' and 'morally active' dispositions correspond to the 'patient-centred' element of 'PERSON'. By answering the questions in the right-hand column you are prompted to critically reflect on your decisions and

Table 7.3: Clinical decision-making 'PERSON' evaluation tool (Standing, 2014, p204)

'PERSON' acronym	Answer these questions to evaluate your decisions
Patient-centred	Were different care options explained to the patient?
	Did the patient give consent before the intervention?
	How did the patient's opinion contribute to care plans?
	If for any reason the patient was unable to contribute to decisions, how were his or her rights safeguarded?
Evidence-based	What patient observations indicated a need for action?
	What corroborating evidence supports your assessment?
	What was the rationale for the selected intervention?
	What research evidence underpins the intervention?
Risks assessed and managed	What threats to patient's health/well-being were there?
	What was done to ensure a safe healthcare environment?
	What procedure did you follow to control known risks?
	How did you escalate concerns if problems worsened?
Safe and effective delivery of care	What knowledge/skills/attitudes were applied to care?
	What prior experience did you have of this intervention?
	How was your competence to give care quality assured?
	How did you share information on the care you gave?
Outcomes of care benefit the patient	What was the patient's/relatives' feedback about care?
	To what extent were desired outcomes of care achieved?
	How do you think the patient benefitted from this care?
	How will you address any negative outcomes of care?
Nursing and midwifery strengths and weaknesses	What did you learn from this experience of patient care?
	How did you justify public trust in your ability to care?
	On reflection, what could you have done differently?
	What are you doing to improve your decision-making skills?

associated care regarding each element of the evaluation tool. In doing so, you will be generating evidence of your commitment to achieve high-quality, patient-centred, evidence-based care. This is important because it can help you to demonstrate your accountability for meeting the professional standards in the Code (NMC, 2015) which requires you to (i) prioritise people; (ii) practise effectively; (iii) preserve safety; and (iv) promote professionalism and trust. In Table 7.4 'PERSON' is applied to evaluate the nurse's contribution to the team's decision-making regarding 'Case study: refusal of treatment', discussed earlier in the chapter (p125).

Table 7.4: Applying 'PERSON' to evaluate clinical decision-making in the 'refusal of treatment' case study

PATIENT-CENTRED

Were different care options explained to the patient? When the 98-year-old lady stopped eating and drinking she was offered an intravenous infusion of fluids/nutritional supplements and the consequences of dehydration and starvation were explained.

Did the patient give consent before the intervention? The lady refused to accept being fed artificially via an infusion.

How did the patient's opinion contribute to care plans? The patient's preference for not being fed via an infusion was discussed by the healthcare team. The nurse advocated on behalf of the patient that she should not be force-fed against her will. The team agreed not to administer nutrients via infusion but to offer fluids/food by mouth and someone for the patient to talk to.

If for any reason the patient was unable to contribute to decisions, how were his or her rights safeguarded? The healthcare team questioned whether the lady had the mental capacity to fully understand the risks to her health and well-being, from her lack of adequate nourishment. If it was thought that she was confused or depressed then it could be argued that the team were obligated to take action to safeguard her health/well-being by feeding her without her consent (she had no living relatives to involve in decision-making). The nurse who had been looking after the lady argued that she was very lucid and on this basis her preferences should be respected.

EVIDENCE-BASED

What patient observations indicated a need for action? The lady had stopped eating or drinking sufficient amounts to nourish herself adequately. She was losing weight and becoming progressively weaker.

What corroborating evidence supports your assessment? When presented with food and drink the lady would ignore it. If the nurse spent time talking to her she could persuade her to sip fluids or nibble on a biscuit but no more than that.

What was the rationale for the selected intervention? To respect the patient's wish to refuse food/fluids via infusion (despite knowing this could hasten her death) in order for her to be allowed a dignified way of ending 98 years of life on her own terms.

What research evidence underpins the intervention? A survey of hospice nurses in the USA reported that the vast majority of end-of-life care patients who chose to stop food and fluids because they felt ready for their lives to end, died peacefully and with dignity within 15 days of doing so (Ganzini et al., 2003).

RISKS ASSESSED AND MANAGED

What threats to patient's health/wellbeing were there? By voluntarily refusing food and drink the patient's life was at risk but the alternative of artificially hydrating/feeding her would be against her wishes and threatened her sense of wellbeing.

(Continued)

Table 7.4: (Continued)

What was done to ensure a safe healthcare environment? Ensuring that the lady fully understood the implications and likely consequences of her preferred treatment option, and the potential benefits of alternative options that were available to her.

What procedure did you follow to control known risks? The nurse had established a good rapport with the lady and this enabled her to assess how she was feeling and whether she felt like accepting oral fluids and food offered on a regular basis.

How did you escalate concerns if problems worsened? The nurse's main concern was to fulfil the wishes of the 98-year-old lady. When the healthcare team were considering feeding the lady against her will, the nurse advocated strongly on her behalf.

SAFE AND EFFECTIVE DELIVERY OF CARE

What knowledge/skills/attitudes were applied to care? Principles of patient-centred care, valuing and incorporating patient preference in care planning. Understanding physical (nutrition), psychological (self-determination) and social (companionship) needs. Applying knowledge to practice by demonstrating ethical sensitivity and collaborative clinical decision-making skills.

What prior experience did you have of this intervention? Third-year student nurse on an adult pathway who had not encountered an ethical dilemma like this before but did have previous healthcare assistant experience in mental health.

How was your competence to give care quality assured? The student was mentored and supervised by registered nurses and her clinical competence in caring for patients was formally scrutinised and evaluated in summative practice assessments.

How did you share information on the care you gave? The student told the healthcare team what she had learnt from the patient and recorded her interventions in the care plan. She also kept a reflective journal of her understanding of acquiring and applying clinical decision-making skills in nursing in her role as a respondent in a longitudinal research study (Standing, 2005).

OUTCOMES OF CARE BENEFIT THE PATIENT

What was the patient's/relatives' feedback about care? The patient was content that her wishes were respected.

To what extent were desired outcomes of care achieved? The patient was not subjected to invasive techniques to extend her life against her will which would have pronged her suffering, and she was supported in achieving a dignified end to her life.

How do you think the patient benefitted from this care? The lady had no one to care for her, she had formed an attachment with the nurse, she knew she had not long to live, and she felt comfortable ending her life in the care of the healthcare team.

How will you address any negative outcomes of care? It is important to document everything carefully to show that the care delivered was justified and in the patient's best interest. It is illegal to assist a person to commit suicide and there is a 'fine line' between not intervening to prolong the lady's life and what might be perceived as helping her to end it. Hence the importance of continuing to offer fluids, food and nursing care to the lady so that she could decide whether or not to accept them.

NURSING AND MIDWIFERY STRENGTHS AND WEAKNESSES

What did you learn from this experience of patient care? The student nurse learnt that quality of life was more important to the lady than how much longer she might live, and she learnt to be an advocate in conveying the lady's wishes to the team.

How did you justify public trust in your ability to care? The student applied the '6Cs': (i) She showed *compassion* when the lady objected to being artificially fed; (ii) She was a key person in the team who had an ability to *communicate* with the lady not just about her treatment but also her likes and dislikes and life history; (iii) She demonstrated *courage* in advocating on behalf of the lady at multidisciplinary team meetings with senior colleagues; (iv) She demonstrated *competence* in encouraging the lady to sip fluids, nibble at food and attend to hygiene/skin care needs; (v) She showed a *commitment* to including patient preferences in the care plan; and (vi) She applied principles of sensitive end-of-life *care* in offering comfort and companionship to the lady.

On reflection, what could you have done differently? As far as this patient was concerned the student felt that she had done the right thing because it was what the lady wanted, and she felt it would have been uncaring to force-feed her against her will. Perhaps the student might have considered ways to stimulate the lady's appetite and assess other possible causes of anorexia.

What are you doing to improve decision-making skills? The student was a participant in a research project investigating the development of nurses' clinical decision-making skills. This prompted her to reflect upon and learn from decisions she made.

The above example of applying the 'PERSON' evaluation tool illustrates its potential usefulness as a framework with which to evaluate nurses' clinical decision-making and the quality of care given to patients. Using 'PERSON' will therefore help you to develop and demonstrate the required NMC competence in this respect as presented at the start of this chapter (Domain 3: Nursing practice and decision-making – Item 10).

Activity 7.11 *Reflection*

One of the main recommendations of the Francis Report (2013) was for health professionals to exercise 'a duty of candour', which means to be open, honest and transparent about the quality of care patients receive and taking action to address any concerns patients, relatives, carers or other service users may have. It is therefore important that you are able to demonstrate an ability to critically evaluate the care you give. Please use the 'PERSON' evaluation tool as a framework to evaluate patient care that you have contributed to.

As this is based on your own reflections, there is no outline answer at the end of the chapter.

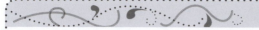

Chapter summary

This chapter has described ten perceptions of clinical decision-making in nursing (collaborative, experience and intuition, confidence, systematic, prioritising, observation, standardised, reflective, ethical sensitivity, accountability) derived from researching nursing students' development of decision-making skills. The ten perceptions of clinical decision-making were related to, and shown to complement, the different kinds of evidence influencing practice and dispositions of the evidence-based nurse (described in Chapter 1). Case studies and scenarios from different nursing pathways were presented giving a context to explore the application of clinical decision-making skills in evidence-based nursing. A high level of patient contact gives nurses many decision-making opportunities regarding planned care, unplanned 'on-the-spot' responses, and contingency plans applied in emergency situations. Sometimes mistakes are made and patients receive poor care. Hence, it is important to evaluate and take action to improve the quality of care. A 'PERSON' evaluation tool was presented with which to evaluate clinical decision-making in evidence-based nursing. It was recommended as a useful framework for you to evaluate your clinical decision-making and to demonstrate your commitment in achieving high standards of patient-centred evidence-based nursing.

Activities: Brief outline answers

Activity 7.1: Critical thinking (page 115)

Dispositions of the evidence-based nurse	Perceptions of clinical decision-making relating to the dispositions	Examples in case study of linking the dispositions and perceptions
• Other regarding	Collaborative, observation	Supporting patient's wife, communicating with theatre team.
• Engaged with self	Experience and intuition, confidence	Use of self to make a difference in caring for others.
• Questioning	Prioritising, systematic	Assessing that there was time to address patient's wife's needs.
• Reflective	Reflective, observation	Judging that offering wife support in this way was appropriate.
• Reflexive	Accountability, reflective	Evaluating effectiveness of care using patient's wife's feedback.
• Creative thinker	Experience and intuition, reflective	Enabling wife to go to the theatre and creating space for her to talk.
• Critical thinker	Systematic, standardised	Applying principles of therapeutic communication with patient's wife.
• Morally active	Ethical sensitivity, collaborative	Recognising and acting on a duty of care to patient's wife.

Activity 7.2: Reflection (page 116)

In reflecting on whether the ten identified perceptions of clinical decision-making skills apply equally to planned versus unplanned decisions, you might have concluded as follows.

- All ten perceptions may apply to both planned and unplanned decisions.
- Standardised decisions more closely relate to planned nursing care, but there is also a standardised option to deal with unplanned situations that you don't feel competent to deal with – that is, to get help from an experienced nurse to maximise safe outcomes for patients.
- Experience and intuition more closely relate to unplanned nursing care, but it is also useful to develop intuitive senses in judging whether planned care really suits individual patients.

Activity 7.3: Research and finding out (page 117)

In reflecting on whether any of the ten perceptions of clinical decision-making skills should be applied in all situations (planned, unplanned or emergency) you might have identified:

- accountability – as all decisions have to be justifiable and defensible;
- ethical sensitivity – as all decisions should be in the patients' best interests;
- observation – to accurately assess patients and evaluate outcomes of care;
- prioritising – to identify and control perceived risks to patients' well-being.

Activity 7.5: Decision-making (page 121)

In applying the Activities of Living model to do a risk assessment of, and to manage someone having, a significant 'grand mal' epileptic seizure (fit) you may have identified the following:

- maintaining a safe environment – remove objects or furniture that may cause injury;
- communicating – assure person that someone will stay with them to ensure that they are safe;
- breathing – loosen collar, place the person on side to prevent tongue obstructing airway;
- eating and drinking – remove food from mouth where necessary to prevent choking;
- eliminating – understand that the person may be incontinent during the seizure;
- personal cleansing and dressing – enable person to wash/change clothes afterwards if needed;
- controlling body temperature – adjust clothing/room ventilation to assist temperature control;
- mobilising – loss of voluntary movement, so minimise injury from involuntary muscle spasms;
- working and playing – help person to manage epilepsy so that they can get on with their life;
- expressing sexuality – person may feel self-conscious or undignified and in need of privacy;
- sleeping – person may need to sleep afterwards; if so, it is safer for them to remain on their side;
- preparing for dying – any seizure increases health risks but a series of repeated grand mal seizures is a life-threatening condition (status epilepticus) requiring urgent medical intervention.

Activity 7.9: Reflection (page 126)

In reflecting on whether the night nurse could have been more vigilant, whether he was negligent and the evidence that could have helped alert him of the risk, you might have said the following.

- Yes – he could have been more vigilant as it is never acceptable to lose a patient.
- No – he was not negligent as his actions were reasonable in the circumstances.
- The most important source of evidence for the new night nurse would have been the verbal information received in the handover. For example, he should have been told if the young man required constant observation and then he would have been able to prioritise his care.

Further reading

Standing, M (2014) *Clinical judgement and decision-making for nursing students* (2nd edn). London: Sage.

Explores and applies ten perceptions of decision-making skills in detail. Introduces and critiques a 'PERSON' evaluation tool with which to evaluate clinical decision-making and nursing care.

Howatson-Jones, L, Standing, M and Roberts, S (2015) *Patient assessment and care planning in nursing* (2nd edn). London: Sage.

Chapter 10 has a worked example of the 'PERSON' evaluation tool applied to patient assessment decisions.

Useful websites

www.nice.org.uk National Institute for Health and Care Excellence website in which you can search for evidence-based guidelines for many different procedures and clinical areas.

www.nmc-uk.org/concerns-nurses-midwives/hearings-and-outcomes/schedule-and-outcomes NMC website link to latest conduct hearing outcomes.

www.patientopinion.org.uk Encourages patients to say what they liked or did not like about care received to inform other patients about healthcare services (also useful for nurses and other healthcare workers to reflect on their clinical decision-making).

Chapter 8
Getting evidence into practice

Peter Ellis

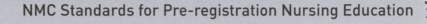

NMC Standards for Pre-registration Nursing Education

This chapter will address the following competencies:

Domain 1: Professional values

9. All nurses must appreciate the value of evidence in practice, be able to understand and appraise research, apply relevant theory and research findings to their work, and identify areas for further investigation.

Domain 3: Nursing practice and decision-making

1. All nurses must use up-to-date knowledge and evidence to assess, plan, deliver and evaluate care, communicate findings, influence change and promote health and best practice. They must make person-centred, evidence-based judgments and decisions, in partnership with others involved in the care process, to ensure high-quality care.

10. All nurses must evaluate their care to improve clinical decision-making, quality and outcomes, using a range of methods, amending the plan of care, where necessary, and communicating changes to others.

Domain 4: Leadership, management and team working

2. All nurses must systematically evaluate care and ensure that they and others use the findings to help improve people's experience and care outcomes and to shape future services.

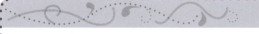

NMC Essential Skills Clusters

This chapter will address the following ESCs:

Cluster: Organisational aspects of care

12. People can trust the newly registered graduate nurse to respond to their feedback and a wide range of other sources to learn, develop and improve services.

16. People can trust the newly registered graduate nurse to safely lead, co-ordinate and manage care.

Introduction

So far this book has identified a number of sources and types of knowledge and evidence, as well as ways of looking at and applying the evidence to clinical decision-making. Knowledge and evidence are in themselves only conceptual entities; nursing, however, is a practical undertaking and it is important this knowledge and evidence is translated into practice. This chapter considers how we might become more evidence-based in our individual and team practice.

Getting evidence, of whatever form, into practice is not as easy as using information we know to have been tested to inform our everyday nursing practice. Before new evidence is adopted, there is a clear need for nurses to assess what is already done in practice and how good its outcomes are – we need to establish what we already know. Once we understand what we already know and what we already do, and once new evidence has been identified, its quality checked and its suitability for practice established, the next step is to understand what needs to be done in order to get it into practice.

In conjunction with thinking about the steps that must be taken for a new practice to be adopted, it is important to work out what might constitute barriers to its implementation.

Kitson et al. (1998) identify that evidence is most successfully adopted into practice when the evidence is scientifically robust, it mirrors what professionals think and it is in line with patient preferences. As well as these issues, Kitson et al. (1998) suggest that the environment of care has to be one that is accepting of change and where there is strong leadership as well as established and reasonable monitoring systems in place.

This chapter will therefore explore some of the psychosocial and practical barriers to the adoption of new evidence. It will explore what might need to be done by individuals and teams to facilitate the successful adoption of new ways of working. The potential benefits of adopting evidence in practice from the point of view of the individual practitioner, the team and, importantly, the patient will also be examined.

A model of the dispositions and influences on the evidence-based nurse was advanced in Chapter 1 (Figure 1.1, p21). This model suggests that any nurse who wishes to act in an evidence-based manner needs to engage with certain behaviours and ways of inquiring, all of which are complementary and supplementary to each other.

Clearly, the adoption of evidence for practice has been at the heart of this book. Throughout the chapter you should try to bear in mind that we have so far identified many sources of potential evidence for practice and that the adoption of this evidence will draw on all of these sources to differing degrees at different times.

Questions to ask before adopting new evidence

We have already established that not all information constitutes evidence because it needs to be assessed for its quality before it can be considered as knowledge fit for practice. As well as assessing the sources and quality of the evidence, it is also necessary to consider how well it aligns with clinical need, resources and skills available, how the workplace is organised and managed, and, most importantly, the needs of the clients to whom, and with whom, the evidence will be applied.

These important issues help to ground the adoption of evidence in the realities of practical nursing. Evidence-based practice for nursing is about dealing judiciously with the sources and complexities of knowledge with one foot firmly in the theoretical camp and the other firmly rooted in practice.

Some theorists claim that nursing is an art and others that it is a science. Certainly, there are elements of both philosophies within nursing practice. If the science of nursing is about understanding the biological and physical aspects of care, perhaps the art of nursing is the ability to draw upon multiple and varied strands of knowledge in pursuit of the best holistic outcomes for our patients.

The activity of nursing is unique because of what it does and the people who do it. What nurses do is varied and tends to be whatever needs to be done. This ability to see the big picture and act upon it (being holistic) and to know where to go to get help to achieve this goal (see the discussion on interprofessional practice in Chapter 6) is what sets nursing apart from many other more specialist care professions. Few other professions can truly claim to stand with the patient at the heart of care, displaying humanity and humility, while simultaneously interacting with other professions to achieve good care outcomes. The potential for achieving this uniqueness relies heavily on the dispositions and abilities of the individual nurse. It is a potential that becoming evidential, in the broad sense we have demonstrated in this book, can allow us to achieve.

One of the first challenges for nurses attempting to adopt new evidence is identifying and over-coming the real (and understandable if not always acceptable) barriers to change.

Barriers to getting evidence into practice

There are a number of barriers to the adoption of evidence, involving a mix of rational and less rational fears and anxieties. Many of us like to return to places and practices with which we are familiar, things and ideas that reside within our comfort zones. Others are always 'up for' change and challenge, regarding the new and unknown as something to be embraced.

Concept summary: personality types

In one of the most frequently referred to models of the adoption of innovation, Rogers (1962) asserts that there are five different personality types.

Innovators	The first 2.5 per cent of adopters are educated, adventurous and risk takers.
Early adopters	The next 13.5 per cent are social leaders, popular and educated.
Early majority	The next 34 per cent are deliberate and motivated by evolutionary changes.
Late majority	The next 34 per cent are sceptical and more traditional.
Laggards	The last 16 per cent are technology sceptics who tend not to believe that technology can enhance productivity.

When managing our own personal and professional development as well as change in others we recognise that not everyone shares the same orientations to change. Nurses, like other people, will adopt a stance to change that is based to some extent on the sort of person they are, their previous experiences of change and their belief in the usefulness of the proposed change and the person proposing the change. Barriers to change therefore arise at a personal, experiential and interpersonal level, and we need to consider these barriers to transition and change before attempting to adopt evidence.

Many nurses do not like change because they understand the practices they are used to and they can predict the likely outcomes of the associated activities; for example, when using a well-tried wound dressing the nurse will understand what a healing wound looks like on changing the dressing, but with a new dressing the look of the wound may differ even though the progress of the wound's healing is going well.

Change takes energy and when people are already working hard the energy needed to undertake change can be overwhelming, especially when the benefits of the change are not thought to include reducing the time and effort that people have to put into their work.

Some of the reasons people do not like to change what they do are deeply seated in our natural desire to be thought well of. For example, if a nurse who has been practising clinically for 20 years is confronted with the need to change a practice that she has engaged with throughout her entire clinical career, a number of questions may arise.

- What is the point of the change when what I do already is good enough?
- If I adopt this change now, am I saying that what I have done to date has not been good enough?
- How do I know that this change will work?
- Do I have the skills to operate in a new way?

These are reasonable questions, all of which may threaten the status and confidence of the nurse confronted by change. These are sensitive issues that threaten to undermine not only one individual but potentially the stability of the team and thereby impact on patient care. There are some simple, but pertinent, responses to these questions.

- Good enough is okay, but the change may make what you do even better.
- What you have done to date may reflect the state of knowledge to date, while the change represents current understanding.
- The change is evidential and the research behind it is well tried and tested.
- You have transferable skills from what you did before which will allow you to adapt to a new way of working.

Resistance to change often arises out of a lack of understanding of the need for change. In these instances individuals cannot see that current practice is potentially not as good as it might be. They may also not appreciate that the effects of the change may outweigh the time and energy required to make the change and that in the long run the change may benefit both them and their patients. The need to fulfil their current obligations takes precedence over making changes because the 'here and now' is urgent and change takes time and energy (Nilsson Kajermo et al., 1998; Hilton et al., 2009) and many nurses feel that they lack the skills to implement change (Rodgers, 1994).

A lack of vision and understanding of the change can stand in the way of individual nurses accepting change. Sometimes this lack of understanding arises out of the inability of a change agent (perhaps a manager or fellow nurse) to adequately explain what they are doing and the likely outcome. There is an issue of communication here that will need to be addressed if change is to be managed at team level.

Often there are issues with the way in which change is rolled out. Some team members may feel the process of change has been poorly handled – it is too rapid, or too slow, or communication could have been better. Others may feel the change is not something they agree with or they may consider the evidence underpinning the change is incomplete or needs further scrutiny.

Consider the questions about change above and whether any of these apply to how you feel about change. Is 'good enough' an acceptable standard for the care which you give or are you the sort of person who always strives to do better? Why is this and what might help you adapt how you feel about change?

As this activity is based on your own reflection, there is no outline answer at the end of the chapter.

On other occasions the introduction of new evidence is hard to instigate because team members have experienced poorly managed change and are sceptical about any subsequent changes.

The National Institute for Health and Care Excellence (NICE) identifies six barriers to change and the adoption of evidence into clinical practice – see Table 8.1.

Table 8.1: Barriers to change (see NICE, 2007)

- Lack of awareness and knowledge of the evidence and changes needed to adopt evidence.
- Lack of motivation both internally and from external incentives.
- Lack of acceptance or belief that the change will benefit patients, that the evidence is good or that it is possible to adopt.
- Lack of skills, or perception of lack of skills, needed to undertake the change.
- Practical difficulties with resources and staff time and continuity.
- Factors in the external environment including the lack of resources and incentives to change.

As well as the barriers to change, there are a number of barriers to the adoption of evidence-based practice that may need addressing. These include the inability to search online databases, a lack of understanding about research, the inability to access research and a preference for seeking guidance from colleagues (Thompson et al., 2001). We help you to address many of these issues in this book especially in Chapter 2 where we discuss access to bibliographic databases and how to search them effectively.

If we are concerned about improving lives and providing high-quality care, we need to focus on the shared value of care. Even if our personal orientation is to be sceptical about the sources of some of the evidence we have to employ as nurses, we should assess the value of the information on its own merit and on the merit of the values that underpin it.

Consequences of not adopting evidence-based practice for nursing

Poor decisions in nursing can affect the quality of life and, indeed, the very lives of the patients we care for. We have identified various sources of information and a number of ways of checking the quality of the information before we accept it as evidence. It is now worth asking the question, 'What are the consequences of not adopting an evidential approach to our nursing practice?'

Activity 8.3   *Critical thinking*

Before you go on to read the next section of this chapter, take a few moments to jot down what you think might be some of the consequences of not adopting an evidence-based approach to nursing practice.

An outline answer is provided at the end of the chapter.

Internationally, nursing is still struggling with both creating and consolidating its professional identity. One of the characteristics of a profession is that it has its own body of knowledge which establishes its credentials and credibility within society. Adopting the broad approach to evidence advocated in this book goes at least some way towards establishing this credible knowledge base, creating and enhancing the identity of nursing as a profession in its own right. This book provides a blueprint for establishing the credibility of nursing evidence while at the same time recognising what is special about nursing as an activity.

If nurses fail to adopt evidential care practices, there will doubtless be consequences for the image of nursing as a whole. It may not immediately be obvious to some why maintaining a positive image for nursing is important. However, when we think about the need for the people we care for to have trust in what we do at times in their lives when they are perhaps at their most vulnerable, the answers present themselves. Care is best provided and best received when there is trust. Maintaining a positive public perception of nursing engenders trust, and this positive image itself derives from nurses being able to demonstrate that their practice is worthwhile.

Within the Code for Nurses and Midwives (NMC, 2015) there is a requirement for nurses to:

6 Always practise in line with the best available evidence

To achieve this, you must:

6.1 make sure that any information or advice given is evidence-based, including information relating to using any healthcare products or services, and

6.2 maintain the knowledge and skills you need for safe and effective practice.

Regardless of our professional standing, it remains the duty of nurses to communicate effectively, in a manner that can be understood, with our clients and colleagues. The important message here is that when applying evidence we should not neglect our core activities of care and communication. Rather, the application of an evidence base to practice should be used to supplement and complement what we do.

Scholtes (1998), when talking about how to gain trust as a leader, suggests there are two elements that need to be got right. The first element is that the leader has to demonstrate he or she has the ability to get the job done and the second is that they care about their staff. If we translate this idea into the evidence-based nursing care scenario, we might readily see trust not only as being a function of the ability to demonstrate care for the people we are nursing, but also as showing that we know what we are doing and why (we have the ability to get the job done).

Failure to act in an evidential manner in our practice therefore puts nurses at odds with the regulations of our registering body and creates questions about fitness to practise. The competencies and Essential Skills Clusters identified at the start of this chapter require nurses to be competent in care delivery and in the improvement of standards for nursing practice.

Theory

Adopting and adapting to the challenges of evidence-based nursing practice is about the constant improvement of care. Within the context of evidence-based nursing presented in this book, the knowledge underpinning these changes is regarded as having been judiciously identified, conscientiously analysed and proactively adopted. Reflecting on the content of these statements, it is clear to see why evidence-based nursing care is a realistic and feasible route to fulfilling the requirements of both the NMC Code (2015) and the NMC Standards and Essential Skills Clusters for pre-registration nursing education (2010).

Acting in the best interests of our clients is a desirable attribute of nursing, although it may not always be clear what constitutes best interests (Ellis, 1996, 2014). Whatever view you choose to take of what 'best interests of patients' means, be this improving their health or maintaining their dignity, what is clear is that no patient's best interests can be served in a meaningful way without some understanding of the evidence base underpinning their care. This is not an empty statement since the evidence base of nursing care is concerned not only with what practices serve to make people physically or psychologically better but also with an understanding of how people experience care.

Accountability

The accountability that trained nurses have for the safety and quality of the care they provide can be demonstrated by the adoption of evidence-based nursing practice. Failure to adopt evidence will mean that nurses cannot justify the care they give (NMC, 2015). While it is true that the obligations of student nurses do not operate at the level of accountability to the regulatory body, they are responsible for their own actions and omissions in the provision of care, becoming accountable for these on qualifying. It would seem sensible, therefore, to adopt a critical and evidence-based approach to practice sooner rather than later.

Accountability is not merely about how we conduct ourselves in practice; it is also about the things we do. Accountability on this level is being able to justify what we do using our professional knowledge, which is drawn down from our understanding of evidence.

As well as our obligations to our profession and its regulatory body, nurses have obligations and duties to their employers. These duties extend to fulfilling our roles as nurses within the clinical governance frameworks established and monitored by our employer and nationally. Clinical governance requirements mean that, as nurses, we need to be able to demonstrate the worth of what we do in working towards the goals of the organisation and in achieving timely, effective outcomes for patients (Scott, 1998).

It seems self-evident that the achievement of safe, timely and effective outcomes for patients is best accomplished by nursing staff who can identify, understand and apply evidence to practice.

Moral imperative

Ethically, it is hard to justify the provision of care that is not evidence-based, where evidence exists. There are many occasions when there is little or no apparent *hard* evidence to support what we do as nurses. This does not, however, mean that what is done to, and with, the patient is unethical. It does mean that as well as striving to do the best for the patient, the nurse operating as a evidential practitioner takes the time to reflect in and on action and adds the experiential learning to their own constantly evolving evidence base (see Chapter 5).

There is a moral duty on the part of the nurse to use more objective and rigorous forms of evidence to support their practice, where such evidence exists (Milton, 2007). This obligation arises out of the special contractual obligations nurses accept on entering the nursing profession. This contract states that we will provide care to the best of our ability and that patients can expect us to do so, not because we are fellow human beings necessarily (although this is also an important factor in establishing our obligations) but because we have taken on and accepted this additional duty of our own free will (Ellis, 2012).

On some occasions nurses may be required to justify the care they have given in a court of law. To this end it is important that nurses can demonstrate, beyond reasonable doubt, that they have provided the care they can both realistically and professionally be expected to provide. Unfortunately, litigation against healthcare professionals, including nurses, is increasing; it is therefore both necessary and wise to ensure our nursing practice is able to stand up to this level of scrutiny.

The main reason evidence is important is that it improves the quality of the care that nurses undertake (Berwick, 2003). Nurses should, and indeed most do, take pride in what they do, and this pride should stem from an understanding that what they do is the very best they can achieve. Providing good-quality care is both good in its own right (it is a duty) as well as being important because of its consequences (the outcomes for patients). The key consequence of high-quality care that is firmly grounded in critical and evidential nursing practice is that it improves not only the outcomes of care but also the patient's experience of it.

Activity 8.4　　　　　　　　　　　　　　　　　　　　　　　　　　　　　*Reflection*

Try to remember a time when you were in receipt of nursing or any other form of healthcare. How did you feel about the care given and was this affected by your perception of the person/people giving the care? Why?

An outline answer is provided at the end of the chapter.

Managing change and transition

Change can be considered to be an alteration to the way in which something is done or the replacement of one thing by another. For example, a hospital or department may choose to change the type of dressing they use post-operatively, or a ward may be remodelled in order to be able to achieve the Department of Health's single-sex ward requirement.

Transition is an alteration in the mindset of the people who have to undertake change (Bridges, 2009). Regardless of the purpose, or nature, of a change, all change engenders an emotional and psychological response from those concerned. Before we go on to examine the management of change, both in ourselves and in others, it is worth stopping for a moment to consider the psychological impact of change.

Tools such as the Holmes and Rahe (1967) Social Readjustment Rating Scale identify that any life change is associated with stress. Hopson and Adams (1976) proposed a model that explains the changes in self-esteem that people go through in periods of transition and captures some of the reasons why people might become stressed – see Figure 8.1.

This model of changes in self-esteem during transition demonstrates there is a level of loss and adjustment associated with all changes. What the model does not show is that the transition through the model is not always the same for all people, or even for any single individual. In fact, Hopson and Adams (1976) claim that different people go through the stages in different orders at different times, and that not everyone goes through every stage for each transition they go through. The stages of transition in the model are defined in Table 8.2.

What these models of the psychological impacts of change and transition tell us is that negative psychological responses are normal. It is important, therefore, that we accept that when we are exposed to change there will be a psychological response, and this is something we should learn to cope with for ourselves, and recognise and manage in others.

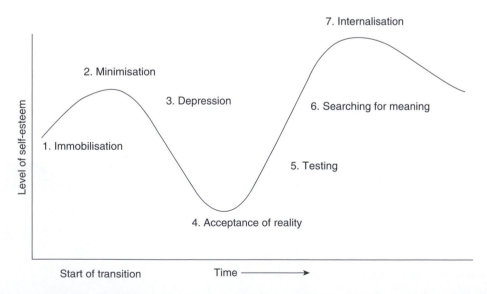

Figure 8.1: A model of changes in self-esteem during transitions, as described by Hopson and Adams (1976)

Table 8.2: What the stages of the model of changes in self-esteem during transitions mean	
Immobilisation	A sense of being overwhelmed and unable to act when faced with a transition. Transitions that are unfamiliar and ones that are associated with negative expectations tend to intensify this stage.
Minimisation	A coping mechanism when faced with change. Frequently people deny the change is happening. This is a common reaction to a crisis which is too difficult to face.
Depression	People may become depressed when faced with the implications of change.
Acceptance of reality	Occurs at the point when people begin to let go of their old state of being and start to accept the reality of the change.
Testing	Begins when the reality of the change has been accepted. In this stage people start to try out new behaviours to cope with the new situation.
Searching for meaning	A reflective stage during which people try to work out how and why things are different.
Internalisation	The final stage of the process during which understandings of the new situation become accepted. The new understanding then becomes part of the person's behaviour.
Based on the work of Hopson and Adams, 1976.	

Managing change and transition as an individual

As identified in the model of evidence-based practice on p21, a nurse who chooses to practise as an evidence-based practitioner must first engage with themselves. This engagement with self is about understanding our own behaviours and orientations. It is about understanding who we are and why we act as we do. One of the mechanisms for doing this that has been identified in this book is the use of reflection and clinical supervision. It is only by examining what we think and feel about situations we have been in, and experiences we have had, that we can critically reflect upon who we are and what motivates us. Other strategies have included being more aware of the nursing literature, especially research, and engaging in a meaningful way with it.

Becoming evidence-based requires the nurse to make two transitions. The first of these involves accepting nursing is about being responsive to new sources of knowledge, new evidence and new understandings. We have to accept this transition is about lifelong learning and continuing personal and professional development, and that change is an inevitable consequence of working in health and social care; indeed it is part of the social contract we enter into as we accept the role of a professional caregiver.

The second transition involves learning to work with the various sources of knowledge and evidence identified within this book, and understanding how these separate types of evidence can be worked into a larger scheme of understanding. Internalisation of these realities is fundamental to both becoming, and continuing as, an evidence-based nurse.

Reasons why nurses need to constantly evolve and adapt what they do and engage in lifelong learning include:

- emergence of new diseases and the understanding of disease;
- development of new treatments;
- changing demographics within society;
- the changing expectations of patients;
- increasing professionalisation of nursing;
- increasing understanding of the impacts of care.

So what does this mean for you as an individual student or qualified nurse? There is a real challenge here in that understanding yourself as a nurse will have a direct impact on how you see yourself as a person. Undoubtedly, reflection – trying to make sense of situations and planning how you will act in the future (Jasper, 2013) – and reflexivity – awareness of yourself and your impact on the working environment (Howatson-Jones, 2013) – are skills that are absolutely necessary to function effectively as a nurse in today's care environments. Employing reflection and reflexivity are essential for consolidating the skills and knowledge that you currently have as well as identifying what skills and knowledge you need to develop.

What is clear from this message is that doing nothing is not really an option for nurses who wish to be both patient-centred and evidence-based. The messages contained in this book point to the need to integrate into our understanding of care not only our own reflections but also the views of our patients and insights from our colleagues.

Activity 8.5 *Reflection*

Even if you are the sort of nurse who employs evidence-based practice methods in your work, this book presents a number of challenges that require development and assimilation if they are to enhance lifelong learning. Reflect on these challenges, especially what they mean for you, and devise an action plan for how you might progress as an evidence-based practitioner.

An outline answer is provided at the end of the chapter.

Critical and creative thinking

Critical and creative thinking, as well as reflection and reflexivity, can be used to enhance both self-development and practice. The skills necessary for criticality and creativity are different, but also complementary, and both enhance the ability of the nurse to become an evidence-based practitioner.

We identified in our model of evidence-based practice in Chapter 1 that creative and critical thinking are dispositions of the evidence-based nurse. Throughout the book we have seen examples of creative and critical thinking under different guises in the identification of sources of evidence, in the processing (critiquing) of evidence and, finally, in the adoption of evidence. But what are creative and critical thinking, and how might they help us become more evidence- based practitioners?

Critical thinking

Being a critical thinker requires that we adopt the disposition of being inquisitive and receptive to new forms and sources of knowledge. It also requires that this inquisitiveness is guided by explicit reflection and reasoned thought processes (L'Eplattenier, 2001). This means enquiry that is both conscious (we choose to do it) and conscientious (we follow a well-defined pattern of thought). Hence, critical thinking is about clarity and rationality of thought.

As critical thinking is about clarity and rationality, it can help lead the nurse from being overwhelmed with information to a position where they are able to logically analyse and unite ideas from a number of sources into ideas (or evidence) that are fit for both implementation and further analysis. The need for further analysis arises out of the questioning disposition that we identified in the evidence-based nursing model in Chapter 1 and the realisation that healthcare is constantly evolving and therefore our evidence base and understanding of care need to evolve with it.

Activity 8.6   *Critical thinking*

Consider how your understanding of nursing has evolved since you joined the profession. Think about what things you found hard to understand – for example, why there is a theory–practice gap – and then consider what you know about these issues now and why it makes more sense.

There are some thoughts and possible answers at the end of the chapter.

Certainly, the notion of the need for constant and repeated analysis through reflexivity and reflection echoes one of the core messages of this book: that knowledge is only knowledge until something new comes along. This underlines the need for engagement in lifelong learning and continuous personal and professional development.

Concept summary: empiricism

Empiricism is based on two related ideas: the first is that all knowledge stems from things we can experience with our senses; it also maintains a place for the sorts of knowledge which arise through research and experimentation. The second key idea of empiricism is that all knowledge is tentative; that is, knowledge is only knowledge until a new way of understanding something supersedes it.

Evidently, critical thinking is not about the accumulation of knowledge, nor is criticality about being argumentative. It is about strategies that enable us to strengthen and deepen our under-standings, and develop ideas and theories with which to underpin practice.

So how can we develop as critical thinkers? First of all, we need to take time to look for and understand the logical connections between ideas. For example, we are frequently told that information giving helps reduce stress in our patients, but have we ever thought about why? Many of us know that stress can arise out of a feeling of loss of control. A feeling of loss of control can arise from not knowing what is happening. So spending time explaining things to patients means they know what is going on, they can make some choices; they feel more in control and therefore less stressed. Next time a patient is angry or irritated by the care they receive, do not jump to the conclusion they are being rude – ask yourself why. This is critical thinking.

In much the same way, we can solve all manner of problems by thinking clearly and logically, looking for connections between ideas and theories of knowledge that enable us to make sense of what is happening.

Critical thinking is therefore about honing our understanding of an issue by systematically bring-ing together threads of an argument in a logical way in order to solve problems or create new understandings (Jackson and Ellis, 2011). A useful metaphor is that critical thinking acts like a funnel, collecting lots of diverse information and knowledge and narrowing it down to some-thing more manageable (evidence).

Creative thinking

For the evidence-based practitioner, creativity follows on logically from criticality. Once we have thought about and understood something, we can decide how we might deal with it. Creative thinking is about exploring possibilities, creating solutions and generating new ideas (Santrock, 2004). Evidently, if we have engaged in critical thinking and thereby understood a situation or scenario, then as an evidence-based nurse grounded in action we need to generate ideas about how we are going to act. Creative thinking therefore feeds into the idea of change and transition.

If we pick up the funnel metaphor once more, while critical thinking narrows a lot of diverse information and knowledge together into evidence, creative thinking may be thought of as more like an inverted funnel, taking the evidence and placing it in among issues such as existing policy, professional and patient preference, ethical considerations and practical knowledge. This broad-ening out in thinking allows realistic and practical considerations to be made about the application of the evidence to practice (Jackson and Ellis, 2011).

Creativity is, therefore, the ability to generate new ways of thinking and/or working. This ability arises out of conscientious exploration of sources of evidence and critical appraisal of their worth. Creativity is also an attitude – a 'can do' attitude that says, 'There is an issue here where my knowledge and the realities of this situation do not marry up. I will therefore find a way to make sense of this situation.' Being creative is a process in which we constantly seek to refine and enhance what we do, taking into account a broader perspective on practice.

Having engaged in critical thinking activities that identify problems and sources of evidence, we can then use creativity either to solve problems or to improve on what we do. The key to creative thinking is the understanding that there might be more than one solution to an issue that is correct, and that the solutions to a problem might vary according to the situation and the people involved.

This idea of the contextual reality of creativity marries well with the central theme of this book. The reality of providing evidential person-centred care requires us to engage with other nurses, other care professionals, other agencies and, most importantly, with the patient, their family and other carers. Engaging with others allows us to see a clinical scenario from more than one viewpoint; it demonstrates the multiplicity of reality and the fact that each episode of care, while often following similar trajectories, is unique.

Being open to critical and creative thinking, therefore, develops the ability within us to adapt our way of thinking and adopt new practices in care. It allows us to deal with change and transition in a proactive and managed way and generates for the individual the ability to be truly evidence-based.

Managing change and transition in teams

So far in this chapter we have laid out some challenges and solutions to becoming an evidence-based practitioner. In this section we will take the ideas one step further and explore how we might manage the process of change and transition in the team setting.

Getting evidence into practice in a team is all about the management of change, and sustaining the impetus of change management is all about creating environments of care that are not only responsive to evidence but are also environments in which nurses actively seek out opportunities to incorporate evidence into their day-to-day practice.

Ward (2003) argues that teams exist to get a job done. Meeting the needs of patients requires nurses to take account of not only the roles of the members of their immediate team but also those of the extended interprofessional team, other teams and agencies and, importantly, the needs of the patients (Elliott and Koubel, 2009).

Lewin's (1947) model of change is often cited in management training. It is a simple model that reflects many of the aspects of change that need to be accounted for if change is to be managed successfully.

Lewin's model is called 'the freeze, unfreeze, freeze model', and is perhaps best thought of by thinking about a block of ice. If you want to change a block of ice from a cube shape to a sphere, then the best way to change it is to first unfreeze it, and then (while it is liquid) pour it into a new mould before freezing it again. This approach is in preference to the 'chip bits off until you get the required shape' which is both time-consuming and subject to inaccuracy in the final result.

Similarly, if you want to instigate change in people, you must find a way to get them from where they are now (the initial freeze stage) to where you want them to be by getting them to 'unfreeze' the way they think and behave, to adapt to a new perspective, and then freeze again in the new way of behaving or thinking. To complete the metaphor this is better than wearing people down in an attempt to achieve the desired change which is both time-consuming and may not achieve the desired effect!

What, then, does this tell us about how to get evidence-based changes adopted by the teams or organisations in which we work? First, there is the issue of identifying what we do now and why (the initial freeze). This allows us to explore the quality of what we do. In order to change, we need to decide what it is we want to change, why and how.

This first stage is all about communication and setting the vision for how things might be and what outcomes we might expect if we decide to change. One example might be the introduction of a new pressure ulcer dressing in the general ward. First of all, we might undertake an audit of the use of such dressings now. This audit might include quantifying how many dressings we use, how much each dressing costs, how frequently the dressing has to be changed, how easy the dressing is to use, the effectiveness of the dressing (how long a particular grade of ulcer takes to heal), the acceptability of the dressing to the patient, the incidence of infection in patients using the dressing and any associated costs of cleansing the wound. This information provides bench-marking data against which we might trial a new dressing.

We may then decide that we want to speed up the process of healing or reduce the incidence of infection-related complications in patients with similar ulcers. A review of the literature on pressure ulcers and discussions with experienced and expert staff in wound management might then be used to understand the options available. Some understanding of the pros and cons of the new approach and some ideas about exactly what it is that we want to achieve will create the vision for how things might be. During this stage it is important to engage all the team in the process so they know what the purpose of the change is and can contribute ideas and insights as well as discuss fears and potential barriers.

During the initial planning stage strategies such as education (Haynes and Haines, 1998), clinical supervision and team meetings might be helpful in overcoming resistance. These strategies also promote inclusivity and demonstrate a commitment to being 'other regarding' as well as exploiting the potential benefits of working with others.

The process of trialling the change – again, collecting data on the variables identified earlier – is the 'unfreezing' stage. 'Unfreezing' is about trying the alternatives and exploring what advantages might be gained and what problems might arise. Again, it is important to include all the team, as they will then be able to contribute to the evaluation of the change. Failure to include the team can create mistrust and fear; it may lead to some people doing things in a different way from everyone else and can derail the whole process.

As ever, the role of the patient in this process is very important. We cannot know how comfortable the dressing is when in place or how much discomfort is associated with changing it unless we ask. Not only does this allow us to assess another one of our criteria for adopting the change, it again demonstrates a willingness to be 'other regarding' as identified in the dispositions of the evidence-based nurse in Chapter 1.

The move to consolidating practice (the second 'freeze') can then occur when the change has been assessed. It is worthy of note that not all potential evidence-based changes to practice can, or are, adopted in practice because of local issues, such as expertise, cost or user preference (Gomm, 2002a, 2000b).

For the evidence-based nurse there is little to be gained from going it alone with a change in practice. The benefits that might accrue from advancing and developing practice can only be fully realised if they are adopted by the whole team (see Table 8.3).

Table 8.3: Managing the process of changing the choice of dressing	
Define the need	Quantify use, cost, frequency of changes needed, healing times, incidence of infection. Establish ease of use and patient preference.
Plan ahead	Review the literature. Consult the experts. Define what a good outcome might look like.
Involve the team	Use team meetings. Consider clinical supervision. Use the expertise in the team. Provide education and training.
Trial the new product	Involve all the team. Get feedback on ease of use and patient preference and tolerability.
Assess the feedback	Decide as a team if the change is worth making.
Evaluate practice	Make the change or stick with what you have; evaluate the feeling of the team and move towards establishing the new or re-establishing the old practice.

Any group of individuals who wish to adopt a 'can do' attitude to the delivery of care must develop together. Developing together is about learning together. Teams that learn together and develop their practice from this learning are said to operate in a *learning culture* (McKenna, 2000). Teams that operate in a learning culture seek out and embrace the challenges change brings. Learning cultures become established when staff commit to lifelong learning; such a culture enables teams to thrive in rapidly evolving environments of care where being evidential allows them to become better responsive to, or even producers of, change and innovation. Cultures develop in response to the actions of individuals within a team and therefore the evidence-based nurse is well placed to influence the development and maintenance of a general culture of inquiry and learning even when he or she occupies a lowly position in said team.

Benefits to the patient

It seems only right to end this book with some thoughts about how evidence-based practice can benefit patients. Throughout the book we have seen that evidence is not merely about the blind adoption of changes to practice identified from within research papers. We have seen that our own experience, the shared experiences of others and research serve as sources of evidence, and that working with others, reflection, the ability to critique research and a conscientious clinical decision-making process help us to process information into something that informs care. We have also noted at various points along the way that the purpose of adopting an evidential approach to nursing care is not merely about ticking academic or regulatory boxes; it is about benefitting our patients.

What is clear is the evidence-based nurse who takes account of the dispositions and influences on practice identified in the model in Chapter 1 will operate in a way that benefits patients in two important ways.

The first is by including them in the process of generating the evidence base – that is to say, taking account of their experience and knowledge. As well as paying attention to the patient's experience, the evidence-based nurse will also be patient-centred in the decision-making process, taking account of patient preference and perceived need as well as other forms of knowledge.

The second benefit to the patient is perhaps more obvious in that evidence-based nursing care is good-quality care – it is care grounded in carefully generated knowledge. High-quality, acceptable, patient-centred care is, after all, what we should all be aiming for.

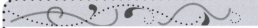

Chapter summary

The process of getting evidence into practice is one of managing change and transition. Reasons for adopting evidence in practice include improving what we do and how we do it. There are also good moral and ethical imperatives for doing the best we can for patients.

In this chapter we have explored some of the strategies we can use individually and collectively to implement change in the clinical setting. The fundamental purpose for the identification and adoption of evidence is quite simply the improvement of practice.

Throughout the book we have presented a series of challenges to becoming evidence-based, and identified a number of strategies and an overall framework that will support the development of this.

Activities: Brief outline answers

Activity 8.3: Critical thinking (page 143)

Failure to adopt an evidential approach to nursing practice will lead to a number of detrimental consequences, some of which are listed here:

- nurse acting under the authority of others rather than autonomously;
- a poor public perception of nursing;
- job dissatisfaction;
- poor use of resources;

- poor outcomes for patients;
- inability to justify what we do and how we do it;
- failure to follow our professional code;
- inability to meet the governance agenda in hospitals.

Activity 8.4: Reflection (page 145)

It is likely that the perceptions of many of us about the people who care for us are based on the impressions we form of them as individuals. This perception will be formed on the basis of their appearance, how they talk to us and who they are. As with all healthcare professionals, the public perception of who they are is based not only on face-to-face meetings but also on their portrayal in the media. This media image is, at least in part, driven by the scandals and other negative events that occur (for examples search for the Winterbourne View Abuse Scandal and Report of the Mid Staffordshire NHS Foundation Trust Public Inquiry). There are numerous other examples where the competence of nursing staff to deliver care and recognise abuse, and standards of personal and professional conduct have made the headlines (see Chapter 7); these most certainly impact on the image of the profession as a whole. There is little doubt that some of these issues of competence and behaviour are linked to the lack of commitment of some individuals to providing high-quality evidence-informed care.

Activity 8.5: Reflection (page 148)

There are many simple personal strategies that can improve your ability to function as an evidence-based nurse. These strategies include identifying simple sources of evidence you can use to inform your practice. You might, for example, set up e-mail alerts from some of the many nursing and medical websites that provide updates of the most recent articles and research in the area in which you work; you might subscribe to a nursing journal; better still, you might start or join a journal club. Clinical supervision is a powerful tool for self-development, as is engaging in focused conversations about care with your clinical mentor. Service users (patients) provide a great source of insight into how care is experienced and what it is like to be ill. Perhaps you might keep a reflective diary that allows you not only to put on paper what you are thinking and feeling but to focus on developing the above strategies to enhance your practice.

Activity 8.6: Critical thinking (page 149)

Critical thinking often arises out of repeated exposure to things. This exposure allows us to start to see connections between issues as well as to explore our thinking and feelings. The theory–practice gap can be a devastating realisation for novice nurses who see it as immoral and illogical. Experience and education enable us to reflect on some of the reasons for it, which include many of the barriers to change we have already identified. This process of realisation speeds up as we start to form theories and understanding of reality and start to see the bigger picture and where things fit into this bigger picture. Applying ourselves to thinking about and understanding our realities is critical thinking; it helps us identify why things occur and place them in a greater scheme of understanding and realisation.

Further reading

Ellis, P and Bach, S (2015) *Leadership, management and team working in nursing* (2nd edn). London: Sage.

See especially Chapter 7 on change management.

Gomm, R and Davies, C (eds) (2000) *Using evidence in health and social care.* London: Sage.

An easy-to-read overview of many of the topics raised in this book.

Koubel, G and Bungay, H (eds) (2009) *The challenge of person-centred care: an interprofessional perspective.* Basingstoke: Palgrave.

One of the few books that considers patient-centred care in the interprofessional context.

National Institute for Health and Care Excellence (2007) *How to change practice: understand, identify and overcome barriers to change.* London: NICE.

This document is simply laid out and easy to read, and can be accessed through the NICE website (see below) by typing the title and first word of the subtitle into the search box on the top right.

Price, B and Harrington, A (2016) *Critical thinking and writing for nursing students* (3rd edn). London: Sage.

A book for student nurses on how to think critically.

Useful websites

www.businessballs.com/changemanagement.htm A management theory website with some accessible ideas on change management.

www.mindtools.com/pages/article/newTCS_82.htm Find an explanation of the Holmes and Rahe Stress Scale here.

www.nice.org.uk The website of the National Institute for Health and Care Excellence.

www.nmc.org.uk Nursing and Midwifery Council (NMC) website where the Code can be found.

www.cqc.org.uk The Care Quality Commission; look especially at the standards by which services are audited.

Appendix
A generic research critiquing framework with additional paradigm specific questions

The first section of this framework can be applied to all forms of research. The later sections apply specifically to qualitative and quantitative research, and ask questions in a manner specific to these methodologies.

Questions that apply to all research

Background issues

Title

Does this identify:

- the type of people to whom the research is being applied?
- the research question/aims/hypothesis?
- the paradigm/methodology/data-collection method?
- the main finding(s) of the study?

Author credentials

Can you identify the author(s)':

- qualifications?
- professional background?
- current job?
- experience of doing similar research?
- conflicts of interest?

Core research issues

The question

- Does the introduction and background to the study identify the need for the research to be done?
- Can you identify the purpose of the research (its aim, objective, question or hypothesis)?

Methodology, methods and sampling

- Given the question, do the research paradigm and methodology chosen make sense?
- Even if 'yes', are there alternative methodologies that might also be appropriate?
- Given the methodology identified (if any), are the research data-collection methods correct?
- Even if 'yes', are there alternative methods that might be appropriate as well?
- With regard to the sample:
  - Is the method of recruiting reasonable?
  - Might the recruitment method introduce some form of bias?
  - Is the sample of the right size?
  - Do the author(s) discuss how it was calculated/arrived at?
  - Does the sample represent the people the study is about?
  - Even if 'yes', are there alternative strategies that might have made the process as good or better?

Results, conclusions and discussion

- Is the approach to analysis of results consistent with the type of data collected?
- With regard to the results:
  - Is it apparent how the data were analysed?
  - Are these clear?
  - Do they reflect what the researchers set out to answer?
- Does the discussion:
  - reflect the results?
  - reflect the purpose of the research?
  - identify practical issues that have impaired the research?
  - identify compromises that have been made to allow the research to proceed?
  - only make claims about things the research set out to answer?
  - explain why the results have occurred?
  - contain additional results?
- Does the conclusion:
  - only discuss what the aim(s) of the research were about?
  - reflect the results and discussion?
  - identify and compare the results to other similar research?

- o   identify and compare the results to existing and potential policy?

- o   suggest possibilities for future research?

Ethical issues

Have the researchers:

- demonstrated the research is necessary?
- gained ethics approval?
- demonstrated concern for confidentiality and anonymity?
- shown concern for informed consent including:

  - o   freedom from coercion (or appearance of potential coercion);
  - o   information giving;
  - o   freedom of choice;
  - o   right of participants to withdraw;
  - o   extra concern for potentially vulnerable participants?

Have the researchers shown concern for the ethical principles of:

- doing good?
- avoiding unnecessary harm?
- respecting participant autonomy (see also consent)?
- respect for fairness?

Additional questions that apply to qualitative research

When critiquing qualitative research, these additional questions, using terms specific to qualitative research, *must* also be considered.

Rigour

- Has the research process been fully explained in a transparent manner that is clear from the article?

Dependability

- Has the study been undertaken in a consistent manner?
- Have all researchers used the same procedures?

Credibility

- Have the researchers checked the level of agreement with their findings?
- Did the researchers check their interpretation with the participants and/or other professionals?

Confirmability

- Have the data been dealt with in a neutral manner?

Transferability

- Does other research appear to support the findings?
- If no, are the reasons for the difference explained coherently?

Additional questions that apply to quantitative research

When critiquing quantitative research, these additional questions, using terms specific to quantitative research, *must* also be considered.

Bias

Have the researchers identified and dealt with potential bias within the study design and execution? Specific biases may include:

- **behavioural bias**;
- **measurement bias**;
- **recall bias**;
- **response bias**;
- **sampling bias**;
- **selection bias**.

Confounding

- Are there alternative explanations for what has occurred in the study?

Validity

- Does the study measure what it says it will measure and do the data-collection tools do what they say they do?

Reliability

- Have the researchers demonstrated that the data collection has occurred in a consistent and reproducible manner?

Generalisability and representativeness

- Where the researchers have claimed the study is generalisable, is the study sample representative of the people they claim the findings apply to?

Glossary

action learning set: a structured group-led approach to problem solving by examining scenarios and discussing solutions.

anonymity: the process of protecting or hiding an individual's true identity.

assent: a term often used to denote consent given for another person, e.g. a wife for a husband with dementia.

autonomy: the freedom, and in some senses the ability, to choose what we will do with our lives and our bodies. It implies freedom from pressure from others.

behavioural bias: bias that occurs when people within a study behave in a given manner because of some underlying reason that usually affects all similar individuals.

beneficence: the ethical principle of doing good.

bias: in the context of research, anything in the design or undertaking of a study that causes an untruth to occur in the study, potentially affecting the outcome of the study.

biographic research: research based on the accounts of individuals who have experienced a particular life event, recounted primarily in their own words.

capacity: relates to the ability of an individual to understand information given in the consent process.

case study: a study that explores individual or small, similar accounts of a phenomenon or disease and may be either quantitative or qualitative.

cathartic interventions: verbal and non-verbal skills enabling others to express feelings.

clinical decision-making: applying clinical judgement to select the best possible evidence-based option to control risks and address patients' needs in order to provide high-quality care for which you are accountable.

clinical governance: a system of audit and other checks health services use to check on and improve their services.

cognitively: refers to the ability to be able to think rationally and provide meaning.

confidentiality: only divulging information that has been given by a patient to the people that the patient has agreed that the information may be shared with, and not sharing the information beyond this group. It is a cornerstone of nursing practice.

confirmability: the degree to which the results of a qualitative enquiry can be confirmed by others.

confounding: occurs when alternative explanations for an outcome in a study are not accounted for. Confounding variables are always independently associated with both the exposure and the outcome being measured. For example, an increased risk of cancer of the pancreas is associated with both smoking and coffee drinking, and smokers tend to drink more coffee than non-smokers.

consent: the process of allowing people to make choices about what they do and what is done to them when they have a full understanding of the facts and are free from external pressures.

convenience sample: a sample taken from a set of individuals who are easily accessed.

credible/credibility: believable; a term used in qualitative research to suggest that the research undertaken actually answers what it set out to answer because of the quality of the way in which the research has been done.

cross-sectional studies: studies that take place within a defined period of time and are used to determine the prevalence of disease or an exposure to a disease.

data saturation: the point during the qualitative research process at which no more new data (ideas, concepts or themes) are emerging. It is at this point that the researcher is most confident that they have collected all the data they can within their sample.

deductive: refers to research that sets out to prove an existing idea or hypothesis – to explore the truthfulness of the original idea.

dependability: consistency in the data collection, if more than one researcher – or data-collection method – is used.

dependent variable: the outcome variable of the study, which occurs as a result of the independent variable having occurred.

descriptive statistics: the use of statistics to describe the frequencies and pattern of numbers with a data set.

embedded knowledge: practice knowledge that is rooted in clinical contexts as they continually adjust to new challenges in addressing healthcare needs.

embodied knowledge: personal knowledge that is rooted in a person's individual identity as they continually interact with others in performing healthcare roles.

empirical: the notion of discovering new things using the senses or, in the case of research, different methods.

essence: the nature of something.

ethnography: a qualitative research methodology concerned with how people interact in groups.

exploratory qualitative study: a study that uses qualitative methods, but does not identify a specific qualitative methodology – often called a generic qualitative study.

generalise/generalisability/generalisable/generalised: refers to the ability of the findings of a study to be extrapolated to the wider population.

generic qualitative study: a study that uses qualitative methods, but does not identify a specific qualitative methodology – often called an exploratory study.

gestalt: moment of insight and understanding.

gold standard: the best known treatment available for a condition, usually based on good research evidence.

grounded theory: a qualitative, inductive research approach used to generate theories in the area of human interactions.

Hawthorne effect: occurs when people respond in the manner in which they believe they should when confronted by a researcher asking questions. The Hawthorne effect can bias a study.

homogeneous/homogeneity: the same – as in homogenised milk, which is the same consistency throughout: there is no cream at the top.

hypothesis: an idea that quantitative research sets out to prove.

independent variable: the causal variable in a study, which may be manipulated during a study.

inductive: refers to the process of developing a theory or hypothesis by first collecting and examining the evidence and seeing where this leads.

inferential statistics: statistics that are used to draw conclusions about the level of association between two or more variables within a study.

informative interventions: communicating skills enabling others to exercise informed choice.

intersubjectivity: shared understanding at a psychological/human level.

justice: acting fairly so that people are treated generally in the same way.

longitudinal: taking place over a period of time.

mean: also called the average; the sum of all the observations in a data set divided by the number of observations.

measurement bias: occurs when something is measured incorrectly in a consistent manner.

median: the middle value of an ordered set of observations.

meta-analysis: a statistical method used to combine the result from multiple studies to provide very robust understanding of the effect of an intervention.

methodologies/methodology: the broad approaches to research that provide the general framework of the enquiry.

methods: in the sense they are used in this book, the specific tools used to collect data during the research process, e.g. a questionnaire.

non-maleficence: the ethical principle of avoiding doing harm, perhaps better thought of as 'first do no harm'.

null hypothesis: the opposite of what the researcher actually expects to find. It is stated in this way in order to aid statistical analysis and to help demonstrate management of potential bias.

paradigm: in the sense that the term is applied in this book, the philosophical position that is taken within the research; sometimes called the worldview.

PERSON evaluation tool: a framework to evaluate clinical decisions using six criteria: **P**atient-centred – **E**vidence-based – **R**isks assessed and managed – **S**afe and effective delivery of care – **O**utcomes of care benefit the patient – **N**ursing and midwifery strengths and weaknesses.

phenomenological: lived experience from which phenomena may be deduced.

phenomenology: a research methodology within qualitative research concerned with understanding the 'essence' of an experience or perceived reality from the point of view of someone experiencing the phenomenon of interest.

probability sampling: the selection of people from a large potential study population that allows everyone the same chance of being included in the study.

prospective: going forward in time.

pulse oximetry: measurement of oxygen saturation of haemoglobin in red blood cells.

purposive sampling/purposively: refers to a method of sampling within qualitative research whereby people are chosen for inclusion because they meet the *purpose* of the study. This means they have experience of the phenomenon being studied.

qualitative paradigm: a paradigm associated with the social and psychological sciences and interested in discovering truths about how people experience the world and why.

qualitative research: research that explores attitudes, opinions, experiences or behaviours through interviews, focus groups or observation.

quantitative paradigm: a paradigm that views the world in a conventionally scientific sense and that is interested in proving associations, correlations and cause and effect.

quantitative research: research that seeks to discover relationships between variables in a statistical way.

randomised controlled trial (RCT): a specific form of experiment that is used in the clinical setting in order to compare the usefulness of two or more interventions.

recall bias: occurs when individuals in a study have to rely on their memory in order to answer certain questions. Such biases are created when people who are ill, or have another reason to remember an exposure, are better at recalling events than people who are not. Last (1995) gives the example of mothers of children with leukaemia being better at recalling having had X-rays while pregnant than mothers of children who are not.

reductionist: a method of trying to explain phenomenon by reference to their constituent parts rather than whole systems.

reflection-in-action: thinking and learning while actively engaged in an activity (thinking on your feet).

reflection-on-action: thinking through and reflecting on an activity after the event.

reflexive/reflexivity: the conscious engagement on the part of the researcher in being open to and expressing their own biases and opinions that might affect the carrying out and interpretation of the research.

reliability/reliable: refers to whether a method of data collection, or measurement, will repeatedly give the same results if used by the same person more than once or by two or more people when measuring the same phenomenon.

representative: in sampling means the people included in the study are broadly similar to the population (or group) that the sample is taken from.

response bias: occurs when individuals respond to a question within a study in a particular way because they think that the answer they are giving is what the researcher wants to hear.

rigour/rigorous: a term used in qualitative research that suggests that the research process has been undertaken in a well-thought-through, explained and transparent manner.

sampling bias: occurs when the selection of a sample for a study may exclude certain groups of people in a systematic manner; for example, an online survey will exclude all those people who do not have internet access.

saturation: see *data saturation.*

selection bias: bias can happen as a result of an action occurring on one side of a study and not the other. If researchers were allowed to decide which participants had which intervention in a study, it is possible that they might select patients they thought would do better in the study or try harder to follow a regime; this would be called selection bias.

study population: all people who fit the study inclusion/exclusion criteria.

study sample: the people who are eventually chosen for the study.

supportive interventions: verbal and non-verbal skills enabling others to feel respected.

systematic review: a process by which various research papers on a topic are identified and appraised for their quality in order to synthesise a solution to a clinical problem.

theoretical sampling: occurs as the researcher builds new theories and ideas from the data they have collected and test this theory by interviewing more subjects to see if the new theory still holds true. Usually only a feature of grounded theory research. Also called 'handy sampling'.

tracheal stricture: narrowing of the trachea.

tracheostomy tube: a tube inserted into the trachea to aid breathing.

transferable: refers to how well the findings of a qualitative study might transfer to other, similar cases. This is generally regarded as having less power than generalisability.

triangulation: a technique used to increase the credibility of research by using research approaches from both research paradigms, or more than one data-collection method. It helps demonstrate the accuracy of what is found in much the same way that providing a longitude and latitude reading helps pinpoint a location on a map.

validity/valid: refers to the ability of a method (or data-collection technique) to measure what it is supposed to be measuring. For example, we know that a thermometer (if placed correctly for long enough) will measure temperature, but it is not easy to be certain that a questionnaire designed to measure quality of life actually does so because it is not always easy to define what quality of life actually is.

variable: literally something that varies, such as eye colour or age. In the research sense it refers to the thing being explored within the study. See also **dependent variable** and **independent variable**.

vegetative state: a persistent coma.

verbatim: word for word, literally as something was said.

vignette: a short case study used to illustrate an issue.

vital signs: measurement of consciousness, temperature, respiration, pulse and blood pressure.

References

Baines, L (1998) Listening to the evidence. *Nursing Standard,* 12 (23): 20.

Barber, C, McLaughlin, N, and Wood, J (2009) Self-awareness: the key to person-centred care? In Koubel, G and Bungay, H (eds) *The challenge of person-centred care: an interprofessional perspective.* Basingstoke: Palgrave.

Barker, J (2010) *Evidence-based practice for nurses.* Los Angeles, CA: Sage.

Barnett, R (2000) *Realizing the university in an age of supercomplexity.* Milton Keynes: Society for Research into Higher Education and Open University Press.

Beauchamp, TL and Childress, JF (2013) *Principles of biomedical ethics* (7th edn). Oxford: Oxford University Press.

Benjamin, M and Curtis, J (1992) *Ethics in nursing* (3rd edn). New York: Oxford University Press.

Benner, P (1984) *From novice to expert: excellence and power in clinical nursing practice.* Menlo Park, CA: Addison-Wesley Publishing Company.

Berwick, DM (2003) Disseminating innovations in health care. *The Journal of the American Medical Association,* 289 (15): 1969–75.

Bloomfield, J, Roberts, J, and While, A (2010) The effect of computer-assisted learning versus conventional teaching methods on the acquisition and retention of handwashing theory and skills in pre-qualification nursing students: a randomised controlled trial. *International Journal of Nursing Studies,* 47: 287–94.

Bolton, G (2014) *Reflective practice: writing and professional development* (4th edn). Los Angeles, CA: Sage.

Brechin, A (2000) Introducing critical practice. In Brechin, A, Brown, H and Eby, MA (eds) *Critical practice in health and social care.* London: Sage.

Bridges, W (2009) *Managing transitions: making the most of change* (3rd edn). Boston, MA: De Capo Press.

Brookfield, S (2005) *The power of critical theory for adult learning and teaching.* Milton Keynes: Open University Press.

Brown, GD (1995) Understanding barriers to basing nursing practice upon research: a communication model approach. *Journal of Advanced Nursing,* 21: 154–7.

Buswell, C (1998) Feeling is believing. *Nursing Standard,* 12 (23): 20.

Cangelosi, PR (2008) Learning portfolios: giving meaning to practice. *Nurse Educator,* 33 (3): 125–7.

Care Quality Commission (2009) *Review of the involvement and action taken by health bodies in relation to the case of Baby P.* London: CQC.

Carel, H (2008) *Illness.* Stocksfield: Acumen.

Carper, BA (1978) Fundamental patterns of knowing in nursing. *Advances in Nursing Science,* 1 (1): 13–23.

Centre for Change and Innovation (2003) *Talking matters: developing the communication skills of doctors.* Edinburgh: Scottish Executive.

Connelly, N and Seden, J (2003) What service users say about services: the implications for managers. In Henderson, J and Atkinson, D (eds) *Managing Care in Context*. London: Routledge.

Couchman, W and Dawson, J (1995) *Nursing and healthcare research: a practical guide* (2nd edn). London: Scutari Press.

Coughlan, M, Cronin, P and Ryan, F (2007) Step-by-step guide to critiquing research: part 1: quantitative research. *British Journal of Nursing*, 16 (11): 658–63.

Craig, JV and Smyth, RL (eds) (2007) *The evidence-based manual for nurses* (2nd edn). Edinburgh: Churchill Livingstone.

Delanty, G and Strydom, P (eds) (2003) *Philosophies of social science: the classic and contemporary readings*. Maidenhead: Open University Press.

DH (Department of Health) (1989) *Working for patients*. London: HMSO.

DH (1991) *The patient's charter*. London: HMSO.

DH (2000) *The NHS plan: a plan for investment, a plan for reform*. London: HMSO.

DH (2001) *The NHS plan*. London: HMSO.

DH (2007) *Privacy and dignity: a report by the Chief Nursing Officer into mixed sex accommodation in hospitals*. London: DH.

DH (2010) *Equity and excellence: liberating the NHS*. London: DH.

DH (2012a) *Caring for our future: reforming care and support*. London: DH.

DH (2012b) *Compassion in practice: nursing, midwifery and care staff*. London: HMSO.

DH (2014) *Department of Health Corporate Plan 2012–2013*. London: HMSO.

Dubler, NN (1992) Individual advocacy as a governing principle. *Journal of Case Management*, 13: 82–6.

Dworkin, R (1993) *Life's dominion: an argument about abortion and euthanasia*. London: HarperCollins.

Elliott, P (2009) *Infection control: a psychosocial approach to changing practice*. Oxford: Radcliffe Publishing.

Elliott, P and Koubel, G (2009) What is person-centred care? In Koubel, G and Bungay, H (eds) *The challenge of person-centred care: an interprofessional perspective*. Basingstoke: Palgrave, pp29–50.

Ellis, P (1996) Exploring the concept of acting in the patient's best interests. *British Journal of Nursing*, 5 (17): 1072–4.

Ellis, P (2012) Rights and responsibilities. In Koubel, G and Bungay, H (eds) *Rights, risks and responsibilities: interprofessional perspectives*. Basingstoke: Palgrave.

Ellis, P (2014) *Understanding ethics for nursing students*. London: Sage.

Ellis, P (2016) *Understanding research for nursing students* (3rd edn). London: Sage.

Ellis, P and Abbott, J (2015) Preparing for revalidation. *Journal of Renal Nursing*, 7 (5): 254–5.

Fasnacht, PH (2003) Creativity: a refinement of the concept for nursing practice. *Journal of Advanced Nursing*, 41 (2): 195–202.

Francis Report (2013) Report of the Mid Staffordshire NHS Foundation Trust Public Inquiry. Available at: www.midstaffspublicinquiry.com/report (accessed 23 February 2016). London: HMSO.

Gadamer, HG (1989) *Truth and method* (2nd edn). London: Sheed and Ward.

Gallagher, R, Fry, M, Chenoweth, L, Gallagher, P and Stein-Parbury, J (2014) Emergency department nurses' perceptions and experiences of providing care for older people. *Nursing & Health Sciences*, 16: 449–53.

Ganzini, L, Goy, ER and Miller, LL (2003) Nurses' experience with hospice patients who refuse food and fluids to hasten death. *New England Journal of Medicine*, 349: 359–65.

George, SR and Thomas, SP (2010) Lived experience of diabetes among older, rural people. *Journal of Advanced Nursing*, 66 (5): 1092–100.

Gerrish, K and Lathlean, J (2015) *The research process in nursing* (7th edn). Oxford: Wiley-Blackwell.

Gibson, G, Dickinson, C, Brittain, K and Robinson, L (2015) The everyday use of assistive technology by people with dementia and their family carers: a qualitative study. *BMC Geriatrics*, 15 (89). Available at: 10.1186/s12877-015-0091-3 (accessed 23 February 2016).

Glaser, BG and Strauss, AL (1967) *The discovery of grounded theory: strategies for qualitative research.* Chicago, IL: Aldine Publishing Company.

Gomm, R (2000a) Would it work here? In Gomm, R and Davies, C (eds) *Using evidence in health and social care.* London: Sage.

Gomm, R (2000b) Should we afford it? In Gomm, R and Davies, C (eds) *Using evidence in health and social care.* London: Sage.

González, J and Wagenaar, R (2003) *Tuning educational structures in Europe: final report pilot project – phase 1.* Bilbao: University of Deusto.

Greenhalgh, T (2010) *How to read a paper: the basics of evidence-based medicine* (4th edn). Oxford: Blackwell.

Haynes, B and Haines, A (1998) Barriers and bridges to evidence-based clinical practice. *British Medical Journal*, 317 (7153): 273–6.

Hayward, J (1979) *Information: a prescription against pain.* London: Royal College of Nursing.

Health and Safety Executive (1974) *The Health and Safety at Work Act 1974.* London: HSE. Available at: www.hse.gov.uk/legislation/hswa.htm (accessed 23 February 2016).

Healthcare Commission (2007) *Investigation into outbreaks of Clostridium difficile at Maidstone and Tunbridge Wells NHS Trust.* London: Commission for Healthcare Audit and Inspection.

Heron, J (1996) *Co-operative inquiry: research into the human condition.* London: Sage.

Heron, J (2001) *Helping the client: a creative, practical guide* (5th edn). London: Sage.

Hilton, S, Bedford, H, Calnan, M and Hunt, K (2009) Competency, confidence and conflicting evidence: key issues affecting health visitors' use of research evidence in practice. *BMC Nursing*, 8 (4). doi: 10.1186/1472-6955-8-4.

Holland, K, Jenkins, J, Solomon, J and Whittam, S (2008) *Applying the Roper, Logan and Tierney model in practice* (2nd edn). Edinburgh: Churchill Livingstone/Elsevier.

Holmes, TH and Rahe, RH (1967) The social readjustments rating scales. *Journal of Psychosomatic Research*, 11: 213–18.

Hopson, B and Adams, J (1976) *Transition: understanding and managing personal change.* London: Martin Robertson.

Howatson-Jones, L (2013) *Reflective practice in nursing* (2nd edn). London: Sage.

Jackson, C and Ellis, P (2011) Whole systems thinking in complex adaptive systems. In Standing, M (ed.) *Clinical judgement and decision making in nursing: theory and practice.* Milton Keynes: Open University Press.

Janesick, VJ (2003) *The choreography of qualitative research design.* In Denzin, NK and Lincoln, YS (eds) *Strategies of qualitative inquiry* (2nd edn). Thousand Oaks, CA: Sage, pp46–79.

Jarvis, P (2006) *Towards a comprehensive theory of human learning: lifelong learning and the learning society, volume 1.* London: Routledge.

Jasper, M (2013) *Beginning reflective practice* (2nd edn). Andover: Cengage.

Jolley, J (2010) *Introducing research and evidence-based practice for nurses.* London: Pearson.

Kemmis, S and McTaggert, R (2008) Participatory action research. In Denzin, NK and Lincoln, YS (eds) *Strategies of qualitative enquiry* (3rd edn). Thousand Oaks, CA: Sage, pp271–330.

Kendal, SE, Keeley, P and Callery, P (2011) Young people's preferences for emotional well-being support in high school: a focus group study. *Journal of Child and Adolescent Psychiatric Nursing*, 24 (4): 245–53.

Kitson, A, Ahmed, LB, Harvey, G, Seers, K and Thompson, DR (1996) From research to practice: one organisational model for promoting research-based practice. *Journal of Advanced Nursing*, 23: 430–40.

Kitson, A, Harvey, G and McCormack, B (1998) Enabling the implementation of evidence-based practice: a conceptual framework. *Quality in Health Care*, 7: 149–58.

L'Eplattenier, N (2001) Tracing the development of critical thinking in baccalaureate nursing students. *Journal of the New York State Nurses Association*, 32 (2): 27–32.

Lewin, K (1947) Frontiers in group dynamics: concept, method, and reality in social science. *Human Relations*, 1: 5–42.

Lobiondo-Wood, G and Haber, J (2013) *Nursing research: methods, and critical appraisal for evidence based practice* (8th edn). St Louis, MO: Mosby.

Macnee, CL and McCabe, S (2008) *Understanding nursing research: reading and using research in evidence-based practice* (2nd edn). London: Wolters Kluwer/Lippincott, Williams & Wilkins.

Maguire, P and Pitceathly, C (2002) Key communication skills and how to acquire them. *British Medical Journal*, 325: 697–700.

Manias, E and Street, A (2000) Legitimation of nurses' knowledge through policies and protocols in clinical practice. *Journal of Advanced Nursing*, 32 (6): 1467–75.

McKenna, E (2000) *Business psychology and organisational behaviour* (3rd edn). Hove: Psychology Press.

McKibbon, KA (1998) Evidence-based practice. *Bulletin of the Medical Library Association*, 86 (3): 396–401.

McNiff, J and Whitehead, J (2002) *Action research: principles and practice* (2nd edn). London: Routledge/Falmer.

Meads, G, Barr, H, Scott, R, Ashcroft, J and Wild, A (2005) *The case for inter-professional collaboration*. Oxford: Blackwell.

Mellor, DD, Whitham, C, Goodwin, S, Morris, M, Reid, M and Atkin, SL (2013) Weight loss in a UK commercial all meal provision study: a randomised controlled trial. *Journal of Human Nutrition and Dietetics*, 27: 377–83.

Merrill, B and West, L (2009) *Using biographical methods in social research*. Los Angeles, CA: Sage.

Milton, CL (2007) Evidence-based practice: ethical questions for nursing. *Nursing Science Quarterly*, 20 (2): 123–6.

Moule, P (2015) *Making sense of research in nursing, health and social care* (5th edn). London: Sage.

Muir, N (2004) Clinical decision-making: theory and practice. *Nursing Standard*, 18 (36): 47–52.

NICE (National Institute for Health and Care Excellence) (2007) *How to change practice: understand, identify and overcome barriers to change*. London: NICE.

NICE (2011) 2010/2011 review. London: NICE. Available at: http://review2010-2011.nice.org.uk/ patients_public/index.html (accessed 23 February 2016).

NICE (2012) *The epilepsies: diagnosis and management* (CG137). London: NICE.

Nilsson Kajermo, K, Nordstrom, G, Krusebrant, A and Bjorvell, H (1998) Barriers to and facilitators of research utilization, as perceived by a group of registered nurses in Sweden. *Journal of Advanced Nursing*, 27: 798–807.

NMC (2009) *Guidance on professional conduct for nursing and midwifery students*. London: NMC.

NMC (2010) *Standards for pre-registration nursing education*. London: NMC.

NMC (2015) *The Code: professional standards of practice and behaviour for nurses and midwives*. London: NMC.

Nolan, D and Ellis, P (2008) Communication and advocacy. In Howatson-Jones, L and Ellis, P (eds) *Outpatient, day surgery and ambulatory care*. Chichester: Wiley-Blackwell.

OPSI (Office of Public Sector Information) (1989) *The Children Act, 1989*. London: OPSI. Available at: www. opsi.gov.uk/acts/acts1989/ukpga_19890041_en_1 (accessed 23 February 2016).

OPSI (1998) *The Data Protection Act, 1998*. London: OPSI. Available at: www.opsi.gov.uk/acts/acts1998/ ukpga_19980029_en_1 (accessed 23 February 2016).

Øvretveit, J, Mathias, P and Thompson, T (1997) *Interprofessional working for health and social care*. Basingstoke: Macmillan.

Parahoo, K (2014) *Nursing research: principles, process and issues* (3rd edn). London: Palgrave Macmillan.

Patients Association (2015) *PHSO: 'Breaking down the barriers' report*. Available at: www.patients-association. org.uk/wp-content/uploads/2015/12/press-release-phso-breaking-down-the-barriers-report.pdf (accessed 23 February 2016).

Pattison, S (2001) Health and healing in an age of science. In Seale, C, Pattison, S and Davey, B (eds) *Medical knowledge, doubt and certainty*. Buckingham: Open University Press, pp14–42.

Petticrew, M and Roberts, H (2003) Evidence, hierarchies and typologies: horses for courses. *Journal of Epidemiology and Community Health*, 57 (7): 527–9.

Pijl-Zieber, EM, Barton, S, Konkin, J and Awosoga, O (2015) Disconnects in pedagogy and practice in community health nursing clinical experiences: qualitative findings of a mixed method study. *Nurse Education Today*, 35(10), e43–8.

Player, MJ, Proudfoot, J, Fogarty, A, Whittle, E, Spurrier, M, Shand, F, Chruistensen, H, Hadzi-Pavlovic, D and Wilhelm, K (2015) What interrupts suicide attempts in men: a qualitative study. *PLOS ONE*, 10(6): e0128180. Available at: doi:10.1371/journal.pone.0128180 (accessed 23 February 2016).

Polit, DF and Beck, CT (2008) *Nursing research: generating and accessing evidence for nursing practice* (10th edn). London: Lippincott, Williams & Wilkins.

Polit, DF and Beck, CT (2013) *Essentials of nursing research: methods, appraisal and utilization* (8th edn). London: Lippincott, Williams & Wilkins.

Rodgers, S (1994) An exploratory study of research utilization by nurses in general medical and surgical wards. *Journal of Advanced Nursing*, 20: 904–11.

Rogers, EM (1962) *Diffusion of innovations.* Glencoe: Free Press.

Roper, N, Logan, WW and Tierney, AJ (2000) *The Roper-Logan-Tierney model of nursing: based on activities of living.* Edinburgh: Churchill Livingstone.

Sackett, DL, Rosenberg, WM, Gray, JA, Haynes, RB and Richardson, WS (1996) Evidence-based medicine: what it is and what it isn't. *British Medical Journal*, 312 (7023): 71–2.

Santrock, JW (2004) *Educational psychology* (2nd edn). Saddle River, NJ: Allyn & Bacon.

Scholtes, P (1998) *The leader's handbook: making things happen, getting things done.* New York: McGraw Hill.

Scott, A (1998) Clinical governance relies on a change in culture. *British Journal of Nursing*, 7 (16): 940.

Sennett, R (2008) *The craftsman.* London: Allen Lane/Penguin Books.

Sitzia, J, Cotterell, P and Richardson, A (2004) *Formative evaluation of the Cancer Partnership Project.* London: Macmillan Cancer Relief.

Standing, M (2005) Perceptions of clinical decision-making on a developmental journey from student to staff nurse. Unpublished PhD thesis. Canterbury: University of Kent.

Standing, M (2007) Clinical decision-making skills on the developmental journey from student to registered nurse: a longitudinal inquiry. *Journal of Advanced Nursing*, 60 (3): 257–69.

Standing, M (2010) Perceptions of clinical decision-making: a matrix model. In Standing, M (ed.) *Clinical judgement and decision-making: nursing and interprofessional healthcare.* Maidenhead: Open University Press.

Standing, M (2014) *Clinical judgement and decision-making for nursing students* (2nd edn). London: Sage.

Straus, SE, Galziou, P, Richardson, W and Haynes, RB (2010) *Evidence-based medicine: how to practice and teach EBM* (4th edn). New York: Churchill Livingstone.

Streubert, HJ and Carpenter, DR (2010) *Qualitative research in nursing: advancing the humanistic imperative* (5th edn). London: Lippincott, Williams & Wilkins.

Thompson, C, and Dowding, D (eds) (2002) *Clinical decision-making and judgement in nursing.* Edinburgh: Churchill Livingstone.

References

Thompson, C, McCaughan, D, Cullum, N, Sheldon, TA, Munhall, A and Thompson, DR (2001) Research information in nurses' clinical decision-making: what is useful? *Journal of Advanced Nursing*, 36 (3): 376–88.

Titchen, A, McGinley, M, and McCormack, B (2004) Blending self-knowledge and professional knowledge. In Higgs, J, Richardson, B and Abrandt Dahlgren, M (eds) *Developing practice knowledge for health professionals*. Edinburgh: Butterworth Heinemann, pp107–26.

Verschueren, S, Berends, T, Kool-Goudzwaard, N, van Huigenbosch, E, Gamel, C, Dingemans, A, van Elburg, A and van Meijel, B (2015) Patients with anorexia nervosa who self-injure: a phenomenological study. *Perspectives in Psychiatric Care*, 51: 63–70.

Virdee, SK, Greenfield, SM, Fletcher, K, McManus, RJ and Mant, J (2015) Patients' views about taking a polypill to manage cardiovascular risk: a qualitative study in primary care. *British Journal of General Practice*, 65: e447–e453.

Ward, A (2003) Managing the team. In Seden, J and Reynolds, J (eds) *Managing care in practice*. London: Routledge, pp33–56.

West, L, Alheit, P, Anderson, AS and Merrill, B (eds) (2007) *Using biographical and life history approaches in the study of adult and lifelong learning: European perspectives*. Frankfurt am Main: Peter Lang.

Williams, G, Dean, P and Williams, E (2009) Do nurses really care? Confirming the stereotype with a case control study. *British Journal of Nursing*, 18 (3): 162–5.

Williamson, GR, Bellman, L and Webster, J (2012) *Action research in nursing and healthcare*. London: Sage.

Index